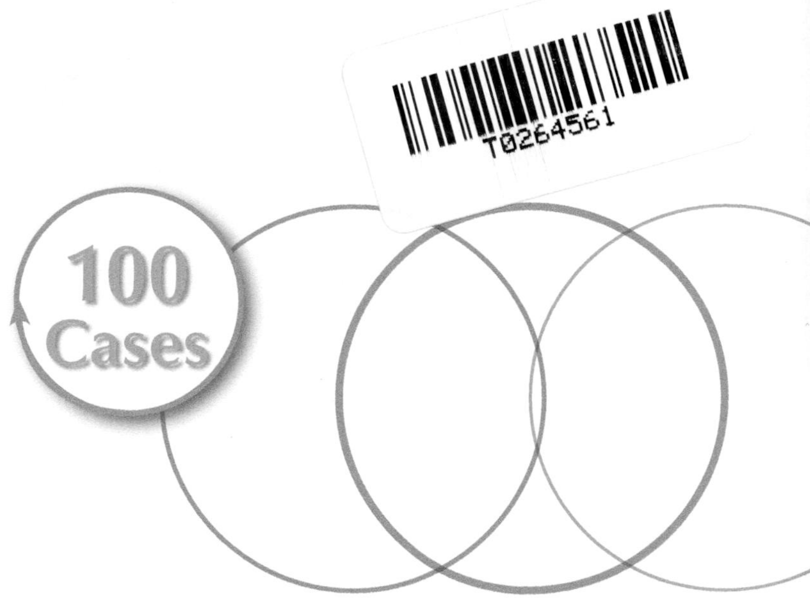

in UK Paramedic Practice

Pre-hospital care plays an increasingly important part in contemporary healthcare delivery and the skills of paramedics, emergency medical technicians and emergency care assistants are a vital part of this. This casebook supports readers to develop the necessary assessment and decision-making skills they need in order to effectively manage a variety of cases typically seen in UK paramedic practice.

100 Cases in UK Paramedic Practice allows for learning and revision through 100 scenarios which aim to encompass cases that may be seen in daily practice. The book covers scenarios that can occur at any moment of the day, from an ambulance shift to primary care settings to event standby duties. The bite-size structure of this book allows the reader to focus on body systems or random case scenarios, depending on their preference.

This is an essential, evidence-based guide for students of pre-hospital care and a useful reference for qualified staff as a source of continued professional development or as a revision tool.

Christoph Schroth is a Lecturer in Paramedic Science and a Paramedic with a BA in Emergency and Disaster Management, as well as a postgraduate certificate in remote and offshore medicine. His experience ranges from the ambulance service sector to remote and offshore medicine in various environments.

Peter Phillips is a Lecturer in Paramedic Science and a Specialist Paramedic in Emergency and Urgent Care. He has worked within numerous healthcare trusts before becoming a lecturer and is now undertaking a PhD studying resilience of paramedics within the UK NHS ambulance service.

100 CASES IN HEALTHCARE

Available titles include:

100 Cases in UK Paramedic Practice
Christoph Schroth and Peter Phillips

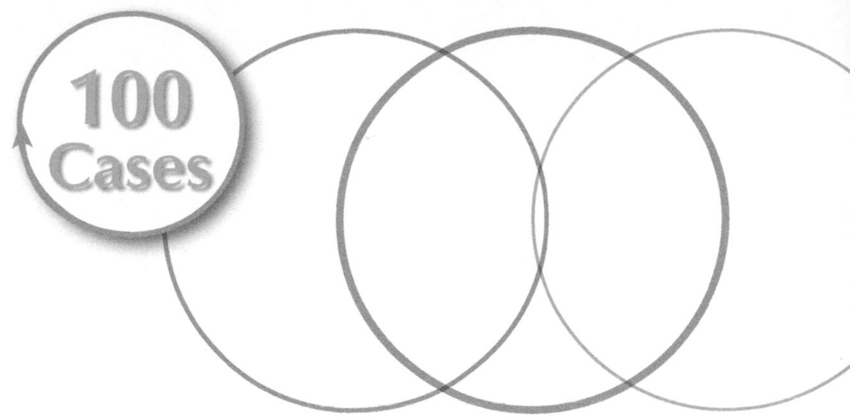

in UK Paramedic Practice

Christoph Schroth and
Peter Phillips

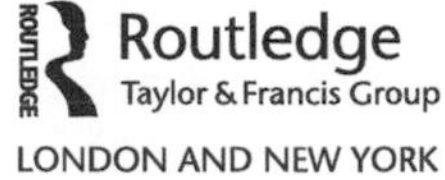

LONDON AND NEW YORK

First published 2019
by Routledge
2 Park Square, Milton Park, Abingdon, Oxon OX14 4RN

and by Routledge
711 Third Avenue, New York, NY 10017

Routledge is an imprint of the Taylor & Francis Group, an informa business

British Library Cataloguing-in-Publication Data
A catalogue record for this book is available from the British Library

Library of Congress Cataloging-in-Publication Data
Names: Schroth, Christoph, author. | Phillips, Peter, 1985- author.
Title: 100 cases in UK paramedic science / Christoph Schroth and Peter Phillips.
Other titles: One hundred cases in UK paramedic science | 100 cases in healthcare.
Description: Abingdon, Oxon ; New York, NY : Routledge, 2019. | Series: 100 cases in healthcare
Identifiers: LCCN 2018024843| ISBN 9781138592810 (hardback) | ISBN 9781138592827 (pbk.) | ISBN 9780429489778 (ebook)
Subjects: | MESH: Emergency Treatment | United Kingdom | Case Reports
Classification: LCC RA645.7.U55 | NLM WB 105 | DDC 616.02/50941—dc23
LC record available at https://lccn.loc.gov/2018024843

ISBN: 978-1-138-59281-0 (hbk)
ISBN: 978-1-138-59282-7 (pbk)
ISBN: 978-0-429-48977-8 (ebk)

Typeset in Bembo
by Swales & Willis Ltd, Exeter, Devon, UK

CONTENTS

CONTENTS

ACKNOWLEDGEMENTS

The authors would like to thank Alison Trinder and Iain Darby for their help with coming up with case ideas and scenarios.

PREFACE

Pre-hospital care, although it is not a new field, has gained significant momentum in recent decades, particularly pertaining to developments within the ambulance service. The evolving role of the paramedic from the short course route towards degree education, in order to meet the exceeding demands on autonomous clinical decision-making and a shift from a focus only in emergency care towards a significant amount of primary healthcare work, mental health cases and availability of new technologies, such as point-of-care testing, has made it necessary for providers and training providers alike to adapt. The aim of this casebook is to allow for self-paced and self-directed learning in a concise and reasonably brief fashion, making it possible to refresh and update knowledge, without the need to set aside hours of reading and dozens of pages to do so. Case-based learning is inherent to many levels of medical education, from first aid to practice sessions within clinical skills labs by healthcare professionals of all levels, because it allows the learner to practise for challenges as they are encountered in practice. Therefore, it is only logical to continue with this approach and build case studies that can do the same for the modern-day paramedic, with a focus on practice within the UK. Every case that follows has been written to address a different challenge, problem or consideration, thus not simply making every case a stereotypical ambulance service incident, e.g. you have been called to a man who collapsed in the street; describe your management of this patient.

History taking is based on two well-established models within the ambulance service: The Medical Model and the AMPLE (CRENSON) model: allergies, medication, past medical history (cardiac, respiratory, endocrine, neurological, surgical, occupation, natal), last meal and urinary output, events leading up to the call to the ambulance service. Both are well known, but the choice is generally up to the healthcare provider and based on personal preference or familiarity. To allow for users of both models to be able to benefit from this book, both are being utilised and have been randomly assigned to the following 100 cases.

THE ASSESSMENT AND HISTORY-TAKING STRUCTURE OF THIS BOOK

To allow for a wide readership for these case studies there had to be a balance across all the methods of approach to the acutely ill patient and obtaining their medical history that are currently being utilised in practice. As such, the explanations below should provide a good overview of the structure being followed in the following 100 cases.

The primary survey and initial scene approach

Initial patient assessment on arrival at the patient's side generally involves the same steps, but with varying angles of approach and detail, depending on personal preferences and educational institution where the practitioner was taught. For the purposes of the cases that follow, the primary survey refers to the assessment of the following areas:

- Scene safety, rescuer and patient safety;
- Check for catastrophic haemorrhage;
- Consideration for c-spine injury (and immobilisation needs during treatment);
- Level of alertness/consciousness (based on the AVPU model);
- Airway (opening technique based on c-spine injury concerns and to assess patency);
- Breathing (depth and efficacy with or without auscultation);
- Circulation (presence of central and/or peripheral pulses);
- Decision and disposal (is there an immediate need for evacuation? How will the patient be evacuated?).

History-taking structures and models

Many different models of history taking currently exist; two of the most commonly used models are used in this book: the AMPLE (CRENSON) model and the Medical Model.

AMPLE (CRENSON)

A—allergies

M—medication

P—past/pertinent medical history

C—cardiac

R—respiratory

E—endocrine

N—neurological

S—surgical

O—occupation

N—natal

L—last input and output (last meal, last fluid intake, last urine output and bowel movement)

E—events that led up to the call to the ambulance service today

The Medical Model

The Medical Model is widely used across healthcare professions within the UK as an alternative to the AMPLE model.

HPC—history of presenting complaint

An exploration of the patient's chief complaint or problem through questions would typically focus on the system(s) that are relevant to the presenting problem(s).

If pain is present you could use two mnemonics to assess the nature of the pain: OPQRST and SOCRATES:

OPQRST

O—onset

P—provoking/palliating factors

Q—quality

R—radiation

S—sore

T—timings

SOCRATES

S—site

O—onset

C—character

R—radiation

A—associated symptoms

T—timings

E —exacerbating/relieving factors

S—score

PMH—past medical history

Including operations, hospital admissions and ongoing medical conditions.

DHx—drug history

Any prescribed, over-the-counter or alternative medicines.

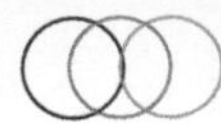

Allergies

Any allergies to food, medication or materials (e.g. latex)

SHx—social history

Including but not limited to:

- How the illness may affect the patient;
- Patient's ability to undertake activities of daily living;
- Social support;
- Occupation;
- Hobbies;
- Alcohol and drug use;
- Smoking.

FHx—family history

Diseases that run in the family, as relevant to the presenting complaint.

ROS—review of systems

An opportunity to ask questions about other body systems to ensure that nothing has been missed and an opportunity to summarise your understanding of the issue to the patient for clarification.

ABBREVIATIONS

5/7	5 days
2/12	2 months
2/52	2 weeks
AAA	abdominal aortic aneurysm
AED	automated external defibrillator
AF	atrial fibrillation
AVPU	alert, voice, pain, unresponsive
AMI	acute myocardial infarction
BP	blood pressure
BNF	*British National Formulary*
C/O	complaining of
CPD	continuous professional development
CPR	cardiopulmonary resuscitation
CRP	C-reactive protein
CRT	capillary refill time
CT	computed tomography
CTPA	computed tomography pulmonary angiogram/angiography
CVA	cerebrovascular accident
CXR	chest X-ray
DNAR	do not attempt resuscitation
DNACPR	do not attempt cardiopulmonary resuscitation
DVT	deep vein thrombosis
ECG	electrocardiogram/electrocardiograph
ED	emergency department
ETA	estimated time of arrival
$ETCO_2$	end-tidal carbon dioxide
FAST	face, arms, speech test
FBC	full blood count
FiO_2	fraction of inspired oxygen
GCS	Glasgow Coma Scale
GP	general practitioner
GTN	glyceryl trinitrate
HCPC	Health and Care Professions Council
HEMS	helicopter emergency medical services
HGT	haemo-gluco-test (blood sugar test)
HR	heart rate
IM	intramuscular
INR	international normalised ratio
ITU	intensive therapy unit
IV	intravenous
JRCALC	Joint Royal Colleges Ambulance Liaison Committee
LIC	left in care
NARU	National Ambulance Resilience Unit

NHS	National Health Service
NICE	National Institute for Health and Care Excellence
NPA	nasopharyngeal airway
NSAID	non-steroidal anti-inflammatory drug
O/A	on arrival
OPA	oropharyngeal airway
OTC	over the counter
PE	pulmonary embolism
PEA	pulseless electrical activity
PERRL	pupils equal round and reactive to light
PGD	patient group direction
PT	prothrombin time
PPE	personal protective equipment
PUBS	purple urine bag syndrome
PV	per vaginum
QDS/qds	four times per day
RR	respiratory rate
RRV	rapid response vehicle
SpO_2	oxygen saturation (pulse oximetry)
SVT	supraventricular tachycardia
TCA	tricyclic antidepressant
TDS/tds	three times per day
TIA	transient ischaemic attack
TLoC	transient loss of consciousness
U&Es	urea and electrolytes
UTI	urinary tract infection

PART I

SYSTEM-SPECIFIC CASES

Christoph Schroth

CHAPTER 1

CARDIOVASCULAR SYSTEM

CASE 1: AN ELDERLY FEMALE FEELING UNWELL

It is a Sunday afternoon, 16:07, when you are dispatched to a house on the outskirts of the city to a 68-year-old female who is not feeling well. According to the dispatcher the patient described it as 'feeling under the weather' and apologised for 'bothering the ambulance service' with such a minor complaint.

History

Allergies: None

Medication: No prescribed medication, but took two paracetamol tablets this morning at around 07:15.

Past medical history:

Cardiac: None

Respiratory: Pneumonia 2 years ago

Endocrine: None

Neurological: None

Surgical: Last doctor's visit about 2 years ago after a 5-day stay in hospital for pneumonia.

Occupation: Retired

Natal: Not pregnant

Last meal and urinary output: Lunch at about 12:30, split-pea soup and some bread. Urine output was the same as always about an hour ago.

Events leading up to the call: Been feeling unwell since she woke up at about 07:00. Did not feel better after taking some paracetamol and she says that she has no way of getting to the local pharmacy or urgent care centre, because she does not have a car, so she decided to call for an ambulance as she did not know what else to do.

Examination

A on the AVPU (alert, voice, pain, unresponsive) scale

Equal, bilateral and clear air entry on auscultation

Radial pulse present (between 60 and 90 beats/minute, regular)

Skin appears a little pale, but closer examination of the mucous membranes does not support the initial impression.

Vital signs

HR 92 beats/minute and regular

RR 18 breaths/minute

SpO_2 96% on room air

Blood pressure (BP) 98/60 mmHg

Haemo-gluco-test (HGT) 5.1 mmol/l

12-lead ECG showing ST-elevation in leads II, III and aVF

Temperature (tympanic) 36.5°C

Pupils 5 mm equal, round and reactive to light

Capillary refill time (peripheral) 2 seconds

Questions

ST-elevation in leads II, III and aVF most probably points towards an acute myocardial infarction (AMI) in which area of the heart?

What is the diagnosis?

What treatment does this patient require?

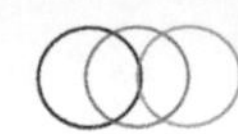

ANSWER & DISCUSSION

Leads II, III and aVF most probably indicate an inferior AMI. One rudimentary way of identifying the location of a myocardial infarction on a 12-lead ECG is by using the SALI mnemonic (leads with ST-elevation alongside the region it applies to):

S (septal) = V1, V2

A (anterior) = V3, V4

L (lateral) = V5, V6, I, aVL

I (inferior) = II, III, aVF

But what is the actual diagnosis—after all she has no chest pain? Silent inferior AMI would be the correct answer here. The exact process is not entirely understood, but it affects only older women and diabetics.

Treatment should follow the current guidelines and include oral acetylsalicylic acid (aspirin), if none of the contraindications are met, intravenous access and transport to the nearest, appropriate cardiac care facility, with a pre-alert en route. Oxygen is not indicated, unless the patient is hypoxaemic. Nor are nitrates or morphine sulphate, because there is currently no chest pain present.

Key points

- No chest pain does not mean that it cannot be an AMI.
- Patients tend to feel generally unwell and do not give the impression of being severely ill. Only careful, thorough examination reveals the need for immediate intervention and transportation to an appropriate facility.

ANSWER & DISCUSSION

CASE 2: PALPITATIONS

During the early hours of a Saturday morning you are called to a 19-year-old university student with palpitations. A staff member from the halls of residence meets you at the entrance and takes you up to the patient's room.

Thomas, the patient, is alert and orientated, but clearly feeling distressed, which is apparent from his wide-eyed look and some of his vital signs:

HR 142 beats/minute and regular

RR 26 breaths/minute

SpO_2 of 96% on room air

BP 148/72 mmHg

HGT 7.0 mmol/l

Temperature (tympanic) 37.0°C

When asked about the course of events he explains that he went out with some of his classmates and that they spent the whole evening in a pub, drinking and watching football. Upon his return home he felt like 'his heart was going crazy' and it started beating really fast, and when this did not resolve after about 15 minutes he asked the reception staff to call 999.

Further questioning reveals that he has no allergies, takes no medication or has no type of medical history, and he mostly drank vodka, mixed with all sorts of things from the drinks menu.

His 12-lead ECG shows sinus tachycardia at 142 beats/minute and is regular with no other abnormalities. Which features of the ECG are of particular importance when making a management plan for a patient with tachycardia (with a pulse)? Is there an algorithm that can guide your management of this patient? What is the likely cause of the tachycardia?

ANSWER & DISCUSSION

Adult patients suffering from tachycardia (with a pulse) should be managed according to the Adult Tachycardia (with a pulse) Algorithm by the Resuscitation Council (UK). Ensure that the patient is being properly assessed and that there are no reversible causes that need to be corrected, such as hypovolaemia, hypoxia and hyperthermia, before looking for adverse features. Signs of shock, and the presence of syncope, myocardial ischaemia and heart failure are not present, thus classifying this episode of tachycardia as stable. A look at the document will also answer the ECG question from the case description, namely the key feature you need to evaluate next, the width of the QRS complexes. His QRS complexes are <0.12 seconds apart and regular, thus vagal manoeuvres, followed by adenosine administration (if in your scope of practice), are the next two steps. Thomas does, however, not respond to vagal manoeuvres and you are not carrying adenosine, so transportation to the nearest ED is your only choice.

The most probable cause of this episode of tachycardia is likely to be linked to the various drinks he mixed with the vodka he drank tonight. Energy drinks mixed with vodka have become a fashionable combination, which may lead to cardiovascular consequences when the maximum recommended doses are exceeded. Asking Thomas about it confirms your suspicions. After a few hours in ED to manage this event he is discharged without further complications of his night out.

Further resources/recommended reading

Resuscitation Council UK (2016) *Adult Tachycardia (with a pulse) Algorithm*, London: Resuscitation Council UK.

CASE 3: SHORTNESS OF BREATH

You are dispatched to a 64-year-old female with shortness of breath while working a shift on a rapid response vehicle (RRV). Following a short response time you are presented with Susan, your patient, sitting in her living room. While assessing her, your auscultation attempts are interrupted multiple times, because she has a significant cough that turns out to be haemoptysis. Susan explains to you that she developed sudden-onset shortness of breath while watching television.

Her vital signs are as follows:

HR 110 beats/minute and regular

RR 22 breaths/minute

SpO_2 of 94% on room air

BP 100/60 mmHg

12-lead ECG showing a sinus tachycardia with T-wave inversion in leads V1, V2 and V3

Temperature (tympanic) 36.5°C

Her medical history reveals no significant information whatsoever.

You attended a CPD session relating to DVT and PE recently which made reference to something called the Wells' score. Could this be useful here or is it unrelated to this scenario? What is Susan probably suffering from?

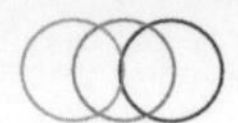

ANSWER & DISCUSSION

The Wells' score is used to determine the probability of DVT and PE, and is definitely useful here, because Susan meets some of the criteria that make a PE likely.

Before calculating a Wells' score, red flags that would have classified Susan as severely ill and requiring immediate admission would have been (NICE, 2015):

- Altered mental status;
- Hypotension (<90 mmHg systolic);
- HR >130 beats/minute;
- RR >25 breaths/minute;
- SpO_2 <91%;
- Pregnancy or giving birth within the last 6 weeks.

She is not meeting these criteria, but does still score points on the Wells' score for estimating the clinical probability of PE.

HR >100 beats/minute = 1.5 points

Haemoptysis = 1 point

Other diagnoses less likely than PE = 3 points

Total = 5.5 points

Patients with a score of <4 points need to be taken to ED for D-dimer testing and further treatment if the test is positive. Susan, however, scored >4 points; hence she requires transportation to ED for an immediate computed tomography pulmonary angiogram (CTPA) or low-molecular-weight heparin, if CTPA is not immediately available.

Further resources/recommended reading

National Institute for Health and Care Excellence (2015) *Pulmonary Embolism*, London: NICE.

CHAPTER 2

RESPIRATORY SYSTEM

CASE 4: SHORTNESS OF BREATH

You respond to a 28-year-old female with reported shortness of breath in a private residence. On arrival you see her sitting on the edge of the sofa in the tripod position, with wheezing loud enough to hear without a stethoscope. According to her husband, she started getting short of breath and used her inhaler, but it brought no relief after about 10 minutes, so he called 999. After a brief primary survey you nebulise the patient with salbutamol and obtain some vital signs and a medical history.

Part of the decision-making in patients suffering from an acute bronchospasm is based on the severity of the distress: mild, moderate, severe or life threatening.

What are the options to determine severity? Which factors should be considered?

ANSWER & DISCUSSION

Multiple factors need to be considered when making this decision. It can be argued that patients, who look unwell, probably are, but this is not all the information required here. Percentile indications regarding the amount of peak flow can be used and are generally referenced within clinical guidelines, but it is not always possible or viable.

However, the way the patient communicates can provide valuable data:

> Mild bronchospasm = communicates in complete sentences;
>
> Moderate bronchospasm = communicates in phrases;
>
> Severe/life threatening = communicates only in single words or unable to speak.

Positioning provides immediate clues, as well. Tripod positioning, such as with this patient, and/or use of accessory muscles are key pointers towards severe or life-threatening respiratory distress.

Other factors to consider are the history and the environment and the clues they may provide: someone known as being asthmatic, previous use of an inhaler without adequate relief, or signs of recent events, such as exposure to food, doing exercise or being exposed to cigarette smoke, could also be pointers to potential triggers or exacerbating factors.

This patient presented in the tripod position, has used her inhaler without adequate effect, is a known asthmatic and is communicating in short phrases, thus classifying this as moderate severity.

CASE 5: SHORTNESS OF BREATH

You are called to a scene where the police had to deploy a CS spray to facilitate the arrest of an aggressive suspect. You arrive to find a 24-year-old male who is handcuffed and sitting on the pavement next to a police car. He is obviously alert and has tears running down his face. Before you approach the patient you speak to one of the officers to ascertain whether it is safe to do so, and it is. He also explains to you that he was resisting arrest after an attempt to steal a bicycle from a local bike shop, and that the arresting officer used a CS incapacitant spray on him once.

The patient is tachypnoeic, has a heart rate around 100 beats/minute and strong radial pulses are present. SpO_2 is at 97% on room air and he says he is in pain and struggling to breathe.

Which specific treatments are required for this patient and what effects are commonly seen following the use of incapacitant sprays such as CS spray?

ANSWER & DISCUSSION

CS incapacitant spray is a 5% solution of 2-chlorobenzylidene malononitrile in methylisobutylketone (MIBK) and is propelled by nitrogen. As it is a sensory irritant, it causes a burning sensation around the eyes and the face, and may affect breathing once inhaled. Bloodshot eyes are generally present and patients should be discouraged from rubbing their eyes. The first step in treatment is to move the patient into fresh air, which the police officers have already done, followed by oxygen administration and flushing of the eyes with large amounts of cool, running water or sterile water, but not with warm water because this may cause adverse effects. Typically, about 15–20 minutes of exposure to fresh air alone are sufficient, however.

Evaluation at ED is not generally required, unless the situation does not resolve and further interventions are required.

CHAPTER 3

ABDOMINAL/GASTROINTESTINAL/ RENAL SYSTEM

CASE 6: DECREASED LEVEL OF CONSCIOUSNESS

The family of a known diabetic called 999 today, because he appears confused and sluggish in his responses, despite having eaten and taken his insulin today. On arrival you are presented with a 33-year-old male, lying on the sofa, interacting with you in a very delayed fashion. The haemo-gluco-test (HGT) shows a reading of 5.5 mmol/l, which is considered to be within normal limits for healthy individuals, but could this still be the cause of his confusion and sluggish responses?

Blood glucose and insulin journal

Monday (am): 6.8 mmol/l

Insulin (am): 4 units

Monday (pm): 7.0 mmol/l

Insulin (pm): 3 units

Tuesday (am): 6.9 mmol/l

Insulin (am): 5 units

Tuesday (pm): 7.8 mmol/l

Insulin (pm): 4 units

After looking at the journal the patient is keeping of his HGT readings and insulin dosages, does this change your treatment plan?

ANSWER & DISCUSSION

Blood sugar values, although generally quoted at ranges between 4.0 mmol/l and 7.0 mmol/l, do not automatically represent the 'normal' range for known diabetic patients. This patient appears to be aiming for 6.8–7.8 mmol/l as his target range during the preceding days, thus suggesting that 5.5 mmol/l should be considered to be hypoglycaemia. Consequentially, he may present with symptoms of hypoglycaemia, such as decreased level of consciousness, confusion, and/or a pale, cold and diaphoretic appearance.

Treatment does not necessarily have to involve intravenous glucose and oral glucose gel may well be the quickest solution. However, this would only be short acting and requires follow-up treatment with a more long-acting carbohydrate, such as a meal or a snack, to avoid rebound hypoglycaemia. After the administration of one tube of oral glucose gel the patient becomes much more active and responds to all questions in a timely and accurate fashion. But what if this did not alter the patient's presentation? In that instance the hypoglycaemia that was initially suspected would have been unlikely to be the cause of the delayed/sluggish responses, and other factors, such as a cerebrovascular accident, should have been considered.

CASE 7: DIARRHOEA AND VOMITING

At 07:00 a 30-year-old male presents with nausea, vomiting and diarrhoea at the local walk-in treatment centre. According to the patient he woke up at around 03:00 feeling nauseated and proceeding to vomit, while feeling very hot and having abdominal and bilateral flank pain.

History

No allergies and no current medication.

No medical or surgical history, other than occasional sinusitis and septoplasty of the nose around 5 years ago.

Last meal was last night at 20:00; most recent output was urine at bedtime and vomiting multiple times since 03:00, with at least one episode of diarrhoea, as well.

His wife drove him to the walk-in treatment centre this morning, as he was not getting better.

Diarrhoea and vomiting are normally not a situation where visiting a healthcare facility is recommended, to reduce the likelihood of further spread of the cause, but this patient has such severe diarrhoea, vomiting, hot and cold flushes and malaise that managing this at home was not something the patient and his wife felt they could do appropriately.

What are some of the key pieces of information that would help you to narrow down the differential diagnoses? Which tests would you consider appropriate other than conducting a rapid primary survey to rule out any immediately life-threatening problems?

ANSWER & DISCUSSION

Diarrhoea is generally self-limiting after 48–72 hours. In this patient, however, there was insufficient time to wait for this to occur, because there were signs of concern present that needed to be addressed (patient did not feel he could manage this presentation at home, due to the severity of the symptoms and the combination of nausea, vomiting, flank pain and diarrhoea).

Before elaborating on the history and potential tests, it is important to remember two of the common causes of diarrhoea: consumption of contaminated foods and side effects of medications (such as antibiotics, laxatives and NSAIDs). A few targeted questions reveal that the patient is on no regular medication, that the last meal was at a take-away restaurant that the patient had never eaten at before and that he ate nothing afterwards. This makes a gastrointestinal condition, such as gastroenteritis, likely because it could be caused by improperly prepared food, which could result in a hepatitis A infection.

To explore the potential microbiological causes, a microbiologist should be consulted for advice and to allow for rapid identification and management of potential cases of norovirus, for example. Urine, blood and stool samples should be tested and a physical examination should also be undertaken. The flank pain is only minor, dull pain and in combination with the urine analysis reveals a urinary tract infection (UTI). Signs of dehydration are also present (altered skin turgor) so an intravenous infusion of 0.9% sodium chloride is started.

Test results show no signs of norovirus, but confirm a case of hepatitis A, a UTI and gastroenteritis. The patient is given antibiotics, oral antiemetics and oral rehydration solution, and sent home a few hours later. The case is also reported to Public Health England (PHE), because hepatitis A is a notifiable disease.

CASE 8: FLANK PAIN

During a shift on the rapid response vehicle (RRV) you are sent to a 37-year-old male patient with flank pain. After a short drive you are faced with a man sitting on his bed, called John, who called 999 after he woke up from severe left-sided flank pain. On examination you find the following:

> Alert and orientated; radial pulse of 98 beats/minute; respiratory rate of 22 breaths/minute with equal, bilateral, clear air entry on auscultation; SpO_2 of 98% on room air; pain limited to his left flank, not altered by position or breathing; pain score of 8/10.
>
> Allergies: None
>
> Medication: Multi-vitamins
>
> Past medical history: None
>
> Last meal/bowel movement and urine output: Breakfast before going to bed after returning from night shift, last urine output and bowel movement before bed
>
> Events: Woke up after about 5 hours of sleep due to severe left-sided flank pain.

You conclude that this patient is suffering from kidney stones, but an ambulance will be dispatched only on your request.

What factors should be considered before requesting an ambulance for transport to the nearest ED? Are there red flags that you need to be aware of? Does every patient with kidney stones have to go to hospital? How should his pain be managed?

ANSWER & DISCUSSION

Not all patients with kidney stones require an ambulance or even hospital admission, unless red flags for cases of kidney stones are present, such as:

- Anuria;
- Pyrexia or flu-like symptoms;
- Frank blood or visible blood in the urine.

These patients need to be conveyed to the ED and NSAIDs or intravenous paracetamol is a good choice for pain management in this scenario. Patients with nausea and/or vomiting may require antiemetics and/or intravenous fluid therapy to manage dehydration, and the need for transportation to the ED needs to be made on a case-by-case basis.

Patients without red flags can be treated at home or in the outpatient setting by a specialist paramedic in John's home, by his own GP, through the out-of-hours' doctor or self-presenting to the local walk-in treatment centre. Recommendations to make to the patient who can be managed at home should include adequate hydration, because this reduces the likelihood of further crystal formation, but needs to be at normal levels of hydration to avoid forced diuresis, which may have negative effects.

Abdominal aneurysms are sometimes confused with kidney stones (in about 5–10% of cases), making a thorough examination with good technique and the medical history particularly important.

Further resources/recommended reading

National Institute for Health and Care Excellence (2015) *Renal or Ureteric Colic—Acute*, London: NICE.

CHAPTER 4

NEUROLOGICAL SYSTEM

CASE 9: 'WORST HEADACHE OF MY LIFE'

A 44-year-old female presents at the local walk-in treatment centre for what she calls 'the worst headache of my life' and is assigned to your treatment room. A quick primary survey to rule out any immediate life-threatening issues highlights no concerns, so the consultation goes ahead immediately.

The headache came on gradually a few hours ago, but it has not been the first time it was present over the last month. Exploring these events in more depth, it turns out that the typical duration is 6–8 hours and presented about 10 times in the last month. Her mother also suffers from migraines and told her that 'the walk-in centre can prescribe some drugs for it'. Which types of drugs are likely to be used in migraines, should that actually be the diagnosis?

Pharmacological options include: aspirin (acetylsalicylic acid), paracetamol with or without oral triptan, an NSAID and the possibility of adding an antiemetic, such as metoclopramide or prochlorperazine.

Are there any red flags that should be considered before advancing to pharmacological interventions?

ANSWER & DISCUSSION

Duration of headaches can be a valuable pointer towards a diagnosis. Tension headaches typically last from 30 minutes to continuously, whereas migraines in adults last between 4 and 72 hours and cluster headaches from 15 minutes to 180 minutes per episode, but in clusters. An association with menstrual cycles, i.e. 2 days before the beginning of the cycle until 3 days into the cycle, also needs to be considered. Menstrual-related migraines are easiest to discover by encouraging the patient to add the headaches to a diary, thereby building an accurate history.

Red flags are a frequently used term in emergency and urgent care and need to be ruled out before exploring pharmacological options. Referral for further assessments is urgently required if any of the following are present (NICE CG150, 2015):

- Worsening headache with fever/pyrexia;
- Sudden onset with rapid increase of intensity;
- Neurological deficit;
- Altered mental status, cognitive skills, personality changes;
- Recent head trauma (past 3 months);
- Headache triggered by exercise, cough, Valsalva's manoeuvre or posture;
- Change of headache characteristics from previous episodes.

This patient is suffering from a migraine and treatment advice from NICE, the BNF and trust-specific Patient Group Directions (PDGs) should be followed. Neurological deficits, such as facial droop, slurred speech and dysphagia should be followed up with a FAST (face, arms, speech and time) exam to rule out a cerebrovascular accident.

Further resources/recommended reading

National Institute for Health and Care Excellence (2015) *Headaches in Over 12s: Diagnosis and management*, CG150. London: NICE.

CASE 10: 'IS THERE A MEDICAL DOCTOR, PARAMEDIC OR NURSE ON BOARD?'

You are on the way home from a conference and about half-way through a 4-hour flight when a public address system announcement is made: 'Is there a medical doctor, paramedic or nurse on board? Please make yourself known to the cabin crew.' As nobody appears to be approaching the cabin crew to offer their help, you volunteer and are led to the business class section of the aircraft.

You are faced with a man who appears to have obvious, left-sided facial droop, which you notice while introducing yourself to the patient, even before conducting any assessments.

After a short conversation with Phillip, the patient, you establish that he is 59 years old and started developing facial problems while eating the in-flight meal about 10 minutes ago. He says he could not keep his mouth completely closed on one side and food kept falling out. When this did not resolve he called the cabin crew for assistance. At this time the cabin crew hands you a medical kit which includes common pieces of medical equipment, such as a stethoscope, pulse oximeter, BP cuff, gloves, glucometer and numerous emergency medications, as well as an automated external defibrillator (AED) and an oxygen cylinder.

You conduct some assessments and find the following:

Phillip is fully alert and orientated

HR 88 beats/minute and regular

SpO_2 of 92% on room air

RR 20 breaths/minute

HGT 5.2 mmol/l

Pupils equal, round and reactive to light at 4 mm

BP 105 mmHg systolic

FAST exam shows left-sided facial droop which includes the eyelid and forehead, no arm drift and no slurred speech, and you note the time when this exam was undertaken.

Are you concerned about the low SpO_2 reading? What is the diagnosis? Does the aircraft have to be diverted?

ANSWER & DISCUSSION

In-flight medical emergencies are not very common, with only approximately 16 out of every million passengers requiring medical assistance on board. However, certain aspects of providing care during these situations may be different to providing care on the ground. SpO_2 readings of 88–93% are considered within normal limits when an aircraft is at cruising altitude, because the pressurised cabin is set to provide an ambient pressure equivalent to 7000–10 000 feet above sea level, rather than sea level. This results in lower arterial oxygen concentrations, due to a reduced partial pressure of oxygen. As such, hypoxia is a concern in most medical emergencies in flight.

Auscultation is considered difficult on board an aircraft, so its diagnostic value may be limited, not only to assess for air entry, but also when taking a BP. Hence you only managed to get a systolic BP, because you based it on palpation, rather than auscultation.

The most likely diagnosis here is Bell's palsy, because the facial droop includes the forehead and eyelid, which does not occur in cerebrovascular accidents. This is not a medical emergency and the aircraft will not have to be diverted.

Further resources/recommended reading

Peterson DC, Martin-Gill C, Guyette FX et al. (2013) Outcomes of medical emergencies on commercial airline flights, *New England Journal of Medicine*, 368, 2075–83.

CHAPTER 5

OBSTETRICS AND GYNAECOLOGY

CASE 11: PV BLEEDING

The ambulance is called to a 22-year-old female with PV (per vaginum) bleeding. On arrival you are presented with Amelia (your patient) sitting on the edge of bed, complaining of abdominal pain around the left iliac fossa and at least half a day's history of PV bleeding.

Causes of PV bleeding are varied and not all require immediate interventions. Causes to be considered must always include menstruation as the first option, but Amelia denies recent menstruation. The presence of abdominal pain could indicate other intra-abdominal problems, such as appendicitis, miscarriage, ectopic pregnancy, ovarian cysts or pelvic infection, but which one is most likely and why?

Before answering this question, here are Amelia's vital signs and history:

HR 94 beats/minute

RR 18 breaths/minute

SpO_2 of 97% on room air

BP 100/60 mmHg

HGT 5.2 mmol/l

Allergies: None

Medication: Multi-vitamins and the contraceptive pill

Past medical history: None of note

Last meal and output: Lunch (about 3 hours ago) and urine output shortly thereafter

Events: Developed acute onset of abdominal pain and PV bleeding about 6 hours ago.

Which interventions are needed and what is the most likely diagnosis?

ANSWER & DISCUSSION

Abdominal pain and PV bleeding can have various causes, but the most likely diagnosis in this case is ectopic pregnancy. This is due to various factors: first, in a female patient of childbearing age pregnancy is always a possibility, until proven otherwise. Second, she meets the criteria of an ectopic pregnancy: amenorrhoea (she denied recent menstruation, but is also taking the contraceptive pill), vaginal bleeding (present), abdominal pain of acute onset (present). Ectopic pregnancy usually presents at 6–9 weeks' gestation, so one missed period/menstrual cycle would fit this timeframe perfectly. Pelvic infection and ovarian cysts are also plausible, but less likely. Continuous monitoring of Amelia's vital signs is essential to detect deterioration and shock as early as possible. Intravenous access should be obtained with a large-bore cannula (14 or 16G) to allow for effective management of hypovolaemic shock and a pre-alert to the ED should be made, as well. Estimation of the blood loss is difficult and should not be used as the basis for judging intravenous fluid replacement volume. Identifying trends in vital signs is more likely to be an accurate indicator of adequate intravenous therapy.

CASE 12: WOMAN IN LABOUR

You and your colleague are responding to support a midwife in a private home, for a 28-year-old female in labour. The dispatch information you received simply stated 'delayed second stage of labour'.

On your arrival you receive a handover from the midwife, who immediately confirms the original callout information and provides you with further details: This is Angela, she is 28 years old and has been in the second stage of labour for just over 2 hours. Parity is zero, gravida is one, contractions are 3–4 minutes apart and her cervix is fully dilated, i.e. 10 cm. There have been no complications during pregnancy and she has no medical history, other than taking folic acid once a day during the pregnancy. She requires transportation to the nearest maternity unit for specialist review and to prepare for alternative delivery options if the second stage does not progress soon.

Delayed second stage: What does this mean? What identifying features are there? What considerations are there during transportation by ambulance?

ANSWER & DISCUSSION

Before going into detail about the second stage of labour, the terms 'parity' and 'gravida' should be defined. Parity refers to the number of completed pregnancies beyond 20 weeks of gestation, regardless of the survival of the baby post-delivery. Gravida refers to the number of pregnancies, regardless of the outcome. Therefore parity 0 and gravida 1 in this patient means that that this is her first pregnancy and first child.

The second stage of labour defines the period between full dilatation of the cervix, i.e. 10 cm, and the delivery of the baby. The diagnosis of delayed second stage in women with parity 0 (nulliparous) should be made around the 3-hour mark since full dilatation, but provisions for this should be made around 2 hours into the second stage, such as the midwife did by calling the ambulance service for support with this birth. Women with parity 1 or higher should be considered to be in delayed second stage as early as 1 hour into the second stage of labour.

Transportation to hospital by ambulance should be undertaken with two small changes to other patient transports: First, if possible, transport the patient with the head of the stretcher towards the rear of the ambulance, that way delivery en route is more easily managed. Second, left lateral positioning of approximately 30 degrees to displace the uterus and avoid compression of the vena cava is recommended.

CHAPTER 6

TOXICOLOGY

CASE 13: STUDENT WITH AN OPIOID OVERDOSE

You and your colleague are treating a 26-year-old American male student at the local halls of residence. The patient is unresponsive, bradycardic with a weak radial pulse and bradypnoeic. According to his flatmates he has been telling them about some white powder he brought back from the USA when he came back to the UK to continue his studies. They are not certain of the name, but say it may have been fentanyl.

After two 400 mcg doses of intravenous naloxone hydrochloride his level of consciousness starts to improve and the bradycardia and bradypnoea are also resolving.

What is so different about fentanyl? What other considerations regarding rescuer safety are so important and why?

ANSWER & DISCUSSION

Fentanyl is a potent opioid analgesic that is approximately 80–100 times more potent than morphine, so very small doses are likely to have significant effects. Two other variations currently available are carfentanil and acrylfentanil. Carfentanil is said to be about 100 times more potent than fentanyl, about 50 times more potent than heroin and roughly 10 000 times more potent than morphine. Acrylfentanil is only about 50 times as potent as morphine, but according to some sources it is supposedly resistant to naloxone hydrochloride. This is not supported by many sources, but should be kept in mind when treating fentanyl-related overdose patients.

Fentanyl powder, in all variations, resembles cocaine and heroin, so it can easily be mistaken for a less dangerous substance when coming into initial contact with it. The particular concern that needs to be addressed immediately with fentanyl is rescuer safety, due to its potency and therefore immediate risk to anyone who comes into contact with it. Personal protective equipment is absolutely vital and must include gloves and respiratory protection. Immediate availability of naloxone hydrochloride, for self-aid and to treat colleagues and other people on the scene, is also essential.

CASE 14: SUSPECTED OVERDOSE

A call to a 19-year-old female with a suspected medication overdose comes in shortly after midnight during the Christmas holidays. You are the second vehicle to arrive at the private house, a few minutes after the ambulance.

While your colleagues are assessing and treating the patient, you attempt to find out more about the suspected overdose, the potential drug involved and the amount ingested. The packets you find in the bins in the bathroom are clearly paracetamol, but the dosage of the individual tablets is not legible. The maximum number of tablets you suspect the patient could have taken is 32, judging by the size of the empty blister packaging, and these are the only pieces of evidence of any substances you can find within the vicinity of the patient. The mother of the patient says there are no other medications in the house and her daughter is not on any medication. At which point does paracetamol become toxic? Does this patient have to go to hospital?

ANSWER & DISCUSSION

Paracetamol overdoses are of significant concern, due to the significant risk of liver damage, peaking approximately 3–4 days after ingestion. The recommended adult dosage is 0.5–1.0 g every 4–6 hours with a maximum daily dosage of 4 g, but how much did this patient potentially ingest? A brief look in the *British National Formulary* (BNF) reveals that the majority of tablets contain 500 mg of paracetamol, with orodispersible tablets containing only 250 mg each. Based on the number of tablets and available dosages, the highest dosage the patient could have taken, depending on the concentration, is:

32×250 mg = 8000 mg = 8 g

or

32×500 mg = 16000 mg = 16 g

Hepatotoxicity may occur between 75 mg/kg and 150 mg/kg of body weight, and according to the patient's mother she weighs approximately 60 kg. To calculate the concentration you divide the dosage by her body weight:

If the tablets were 250 mg each: 8000 mg divided by 60 kg = 133.34 mg/kg

If the tablets were 500 mg each: 16 000 divided by 60 kg = 266.67 mg/kg

Both of these figures are clearly within or beyond the concentration that may cause hepatotoxicity, and hospitalisation is definitely required. Immediate treatment considerations should include activated charcoal, if within your scope of practice, which provides the most benefit if administered within 1 hour of ingestion. Hospital treatment will most likely include an acetylcysteine infusion to protect the patient's liver from damage, and regular monitoring of liver function and her plasma concentration of paracetamol will be undertaken. The National Poisons Information Service (NPIS) and in-house toxicology department will also be consulted after her arrival in the ED.

Further resources/recommended reading

British National Formulary, Emergency treatment of poisoning (in print, via the smartphone app or via www.medicinescomplete.com)

National Poisons Information Service: www.npis.org

TOXBASE: www.toxbase.org

CHAPTER 7

RESUSCITATION

CASE 15: COLLAPSE AT THE BUS STOP

'Ambulance 51, please respond to the bus stop in front of the convention centre for a collapse case. No further details. Police are also en route.'

Upon arrival 4 minutes later you are faced with an adult male lying next to the bus stop, surrounded by a few onlookers and a man performing hands-only cardiopulmonary resuscitation (CPR). You and your colleague immediately take over compressions, apply a manual defibrillator and conduct a rhythm check. The monitor shows a normal sinus rhythm at a rate of 68 beats/minute and the patient has no palpable carotid pulse, so a PEA (pulseless electrical activity) arrest is confirmed and no shock is indicated. CPR is continued. An iGel supraglottic airway is inserted to allow for asynchronous CPR, and an intravenous cannula is inserted for the purposes of drug administration. Now the time has come to consider the reversible causes of cardiac arrest, commonly referred to as the 'Hs & Ts', namely:

- Hypoxia;
- Hypovolaemia;
- Hyperkalaemia, hypokalaemia, hypoglycaemia and other metabolic disorders;
- Hypothermia;
- Tension pneumothorax;
- Tamponade (cardiac tamponade);
- Thrombosis (coronary or pulmonary);
- Toxins.

What methods, tests and interventions are available in the pre-hospital setting to address or rule out these reversible causes? Consider each reversible cause before turning the page for suggestions, ideas and options.

ANSWER & DISCUSSION

Cardiac arrest management can require a significant amount of knowledge and physical and mental input by all involved parties, not just the ambulance crew. Bystander CPR is essential in increasing survival chances in victims of sudden cardiac arrest. Please remember to thank bystanders for their efforts and acknowledge their contribution in trying to save a life. This may have been the first time they ever had to do this and this should not go unnoticed.

Reversible causes listed on the previous page, and which methods, tests and interventions are available to address them, are elaborated on, below:

- Hypoxia: ensuring effective, bilateral chest rise; high-quality chest compressions; providing high concentration oxygen and monitoring $ETCO_2$ via waveform capnography, are all essential;
- Hypovolaemia: obtaining a thorough medical history and history of events leading up to the cardiac arrest is an essential step. Assessing chest, abdomen, pelvis and long bones for signs of significant injury/internal bleeding. Skin turgor, moisture levels and colour of mucous membranes should also be assessed in all patients in cardiac arrest;
- Hyperkalaemia and metabolic disorders: obtaining a blood glucose reading and a thorough medical history are essential. Signs of hyperkalaemia, such as ECG changes (Strings' sign), are late and rare signs. Establishing whether renal failure is a possibility and the history of current medications are essential;
- Hypothermia: a tympanic temperature may not be accurate, particularly if the patient's ears are wet. Consider the environment, not just the reading of the thermometer (i.e. wind chill, time elapsed since the cardiac arrest occurred);
- Tension pneumothorax: auscultation is probably the most reliable way of establishing diminished or decreased air entry on one or both sides of the chest. Tracheal deviation and jugular venous distension are very late signs. Needle thoracocentesis should be undertaken with a 14G intravenous cannula or specialised device;
- Tamponade (cardiac): auscultation during a cardiac arrest is of no benefit. History suggesting chest trauma may raise suspicions. Ultrasound is an ideal way to confirm this diagnosis, but is not always available on scene. Transportation may be warranted to allow for treatment in hospital or via specialist resources (HEMS doctor or other specialist with a similar skillset and equipment);
- Thrombosis (coronary or pulmonary): history of events and previous thrombosis increases the likelihood of recurrence. Consider deep vein thromboses (DVTs), recent surgery, scuba diving and air travel;
- Toxins: medical history, illicit drug use and dosing errors of prescribed medication are all potential contributors to a toxicological scenario.

Further resources/recommended reading

Resuscitation Council UK (2015) *Adult Advanced Life Support*, London: Resuscitation Council UK.

CASE 16: CPR AT THE WATERPARK

You are working on a reflective essay about a cardiac arrest case at a local waterpark that you attended a few days ago and are doing some research and reading around the subject area of drowning. You have already established that terms such as 'dry drowning', 'secondary drowning' and 'near drowning' should be avoided and that 'fatal drowning' and 'non-fatal drowning' are the terms that should be used instead. The definition of drowning by the World Health Organization is also something you have looked up: 'Drowning is the process of experiencing respiratory impairment from submersion/immersion in liquid' (WHO, 2002).

Before actually writing the essay, what are some topic areas, key points, areas of concern or random thoughts with regard to a cardiac arrest scenario that you might have to consider?

ANSWER & DISCUSSION

Resuscitation of drowning victims needs to include a few key considerations, topic areas or adjustment of procedures:

- Rescuer safety is a major concern;
- Removal from the water should be as quick as possible. Spinal immobilisation is not a key priority and the overall risk of spinal injuries in drownings is low;
- Keeping the patient horizontal when rescuing them from the water may reduce the likelihood of it progressing to cardiac arrest (during and after the rescue);
- Positive outcomes are likely if submersion duration was less than 10 minutes;
- Search and rescue efforts should be re-evaluated/reviewed every 30 minutes to assess the risk to the rescuers and likelihood of a positive outcome;
- Five rescue breaths are recommended for adults and children;
- Stepwise airway management should be escalated to endotracheal intubation as soon as possible, to reduce the likelihood of regurgitation;
- A suction unit should be available at all times;
- Hypothermia is likely; heating blankets and warming the environment should be considered;
- Do not use tympanic thermometers in drowning victims, because wet and cold ears will significantly affect the result and not be a true reflection of the patient's temperature'
- Defibrillation in patients with a core temperature of <30°C should be limited to three shocks at maximum energy output;
- Adrenaline and amiodarone must be withheld until the core temperature is >30°C;
- Between 30 and 35°C drug administration intervals should be doubled; once >35°C is reached the normal advanced life support intervals should be followed.

Further resources/recommended reading

World Health Organization (2002) *Drowning*, Geneva: WHO, available at: www.who.int.

Resuscitation Council UK, *Prehospital Resuscitation*, London: Resuscitation Council UK, available at: www.resus.org.uk.

CHAPTER 8

MENTAL HEALTH

CASE 17: SELF-HARM

You and your female colleague (both paramedics) are sent to an attempted suicide case in an apartment block; according to the dispatcher the patient tried to slit her wrists, but managed to call the ambulance herself. A short 3-minute response time and you arrive at the patient's flat. Claire, the 22-year-old patient, meets you at the door, while applying pressure to her left arm with a towel. She leads you to the living room and takes a seat on the sofa. After introducing yourself, Claire is not keen on talking to you, the male crew member, at all. Your colleague Alison, however, appears to be the preferred person for Claire to talk to, but fails to completely open up while you are within earshot. You decide to step out of the room to give Claire a safe space to open up and talk, while staying close enough to provide support and backup if things get out of hand, or the medical need arises, to return immediately.

About 10 minutes later Alison comes out the living room to discuss the situation with you. Claire allowed her to look at the lacerations on her left arm and they are all superficial. She did not allow her to obtain any vital signs, but does not appear to be confused or lacking capacity. She also told her that she was in an abusive relationship until a few months ago and has been undertaking minor self-harm attempts, but never anything with serious intent. She feels like she has nobody to talk to and that she thinks the fact her ex-boyfriend hurt her is because she was not as good a girlfriend as she could have been.

She does not want to go to hospital and you have no doubt about her level of mental capacity at this time. What supporting measures could you put in place or recommend? Can you discharge Claire on scene?

ANSWER & DISCUSSION

Claire self-harmed today, but has no history or clues towards having a specific plan for suicide or significant self-harm. She has not given you any reasons to doubt her mental capacity, either, making it possible to discharge her on scene. However, support should be provided to allow her to manage this stressful time. This could be by calling her mental health crisis team and one of her friends or family who she trusts enough to be with and talk to. The crisis team is only a support service, so they will not actually be visiting her at home, so friends are likely to be a valuable resource. Alternatively, support groups, charities and helplines are also a strong form of available support. Below are some details you could share with Claire:

- Mind (www.mind.org.uk) 0300 123 3393 (Monday to Friday, 09:00–16:00);
- National Self Harm Network–online forums for those who self-harm (www.nshn.co.uk);
- Samaritans (www.samaritans.org) 116 123 (UK & ROI) (24 hours a day);
- Sane–phone, text and online support for mental health patients, families and carers (www.sane.org.uk) 0300 304 7000 (16:30–22:30 every day);

Further resources/recommended reading

National Institute for Health and Care Excellence (2014) *Self-harm*, London: NICE.

CHAPTER 9

PAEDIATRICS

CASE 18: CHILD WITH A RASH

You have been dispatched to a 3-year-old child with a rash and pyrexia and according to the caller 'it could be meningitis'. Upon arrival you are faced with the child sitting on the floor of the lounge, playing with toys and a worried-looking mother starting to give you some information as you enter the house. While this is happening you gain an initial impression by using the paediatric assessment triangle (PAT), which evaluates a child's overall medical status in a non-invasive manner (see below).

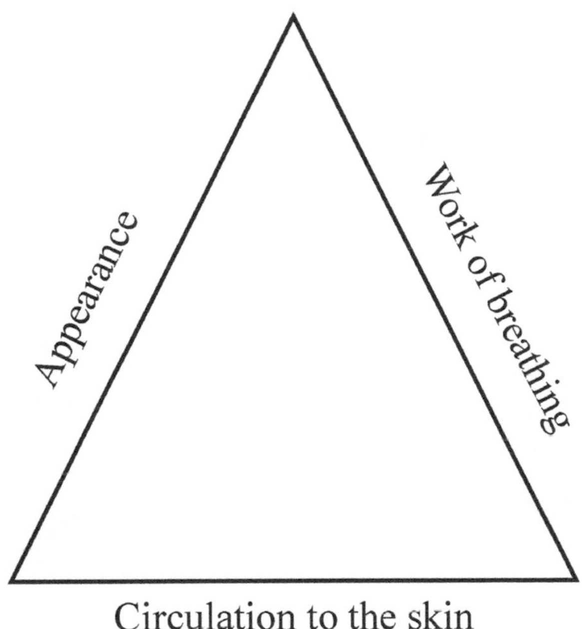

Figure 1.1 Paediatric assessment triangle

The child is showing no deficits on the PAT, thus reducing the priority of care that is needed at this time, and giving you more time to obtain further information and to assess the child in more detail. According to the mother, her son Joseph has had a rash on his buttocks for a few days already, is very warm to the touch and that this is 'exactly what happens with meningitis'. Apparently a recent article in the local newspaper advised parents to call 999 immediately when these signs are present, so she did.

During the physical assessment of Joseph you find no abnormalities, other than a nappy rash and a tympanic temperature of 37.3°C, and the history does not suggest anything that could point towards meningitis.

What are the key characteristics that would have to be present to make meningitis a likely diagnosis and what treatment considerations should be made?

 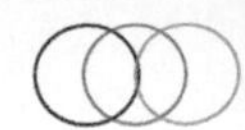

ANSWER & DISCUSSION

Meningitis is not an unreasonable assumption in many situations, particularly when recent cases in the area may have raised parents' suspicions. That being said, there are certain criteria that make the diagnosis more or less likely.

Pyrexia in children is not an uncommon occurrence and should not be considered a key indicator of severe illness. The rash the mother noticed, although not a guaranteed indicator of meningitis is often present as a non-blanching variant. This is, however, not the case here, either. Brudzinski's sign (to identify neck stiffness, which causes hips and knees to flex when the neck is flexed) and Kernig's sign (the inability to straighten the patient's leg, when lying supine and the hip being flexed to 90°) are both used to identify signs of meningeal inflammation. However, these are also not guaranteed identifiers, but a non-blanching rash, photophobia, and an altered mental state with or without a positive Brudzinski's and/or Kernig's sign are red flags for meningitis. Treatment of bacterial meningitis would have to include benzylpenicillin, if available and not contraindicated, and require urgent review and treatment in hospital and a pre-alert.

In this case, however, there are no red flags for meningitis present and this child could be safely discharged at home, assuming the mother agrees with this plan of action. Appropriate safety netting should be put in place, i.e. contacting 111 or 999, depending on the severity of symptoms.

CHAPTER 10

TRAUMA

CASE 19: STABBED ABDOMEN

Working a night shift on a rapid response vehicle (RRV) you are dispatched to a patient who was reportedly stabbed in the abdomen. The scene has been secured by the police and a male in his mid-20s is assessed: he is alert and orientated, HR of 96 beats/minute, RR of 22 breaths/minute and a single stab wound to the right lower quadrant of the abdomen. There is no exsanguinating haemorrhage present. The knife was recovered by the police – a kitchen knife with a 5-cm (2-inch)-long blade. While awaiting the arrival of an ambulance to convey the patient to the nearest ED, you obtain some more vital signs:

SpO_2 of 97% on oxygen, ECG showing a heart rate of 94 beats/minute and a normal sinus rhythm and a BP of 80/50 mmHg. This patient is hypotensive and you have a few minutes until the ambulance arrives, so you decide to cannulate the patient's left arm with a 16G cannula.

The question is: Does this patient require intravenous fluids at this time?

ANSWER & DISCUSSION

Hypotension, by definition, is a systolic BP of <90 mmHg and this patient meets that criterion, but intravenous fluid administration is contraindicated here. This is simply because, in penetrating trunk trauma, permissive hypotension (i.e. allowing the patient to have a BP <90 mmHg) has been shown to improve outcomes. Trauma management guidelines, the JRCALC (Joint Royal Colleges Ambulance Liaison Committee) and various ambulance trust guidelines have therefore been modified to set specific limits for permissive hypotension in trauma patients:

Penetrating trunk trauma: 60 mmHg systolic

Non-penetrating trunk trauma: 90 mmHg systolic

Head injury/head trauma: 110–120 mmHg systolic

The reason for this is the negative impact an increased BP could have on the viability of formed blood clots, which could be dislodged or stopped from forming by increasing the BP of all trauma patients to the same 90 mmHg systolic limit. The challenge with the limits mentioned above is, however, that, in a poly-trauma patient with a combination of penetrating and non-penetrating trauma and a head injury, for example, there is no single best answer for the ideal BP and professional judgement will have to suffice to make this decision. The patient in this case only has isolated trunk trauma, hence 60 mmHg systolic is the applicable indicated BP to administer intravenous fluids.

CASE 20: ADULT WITH BURNS

You are first on scene of an adult male with bilateral burns to his arms. Upon arrival the patient's wife explains to you what happened. Robert, the patient, was attempting to fix his hot water boiler which kept on giving a high pressure warning. After he removed the outer cover and attempted to adjust it a pipe burst and scalded both his arms, leaving him in agony. His wife immediately shut off the water supply, boiler and gas, and called 999. While awaiting your arrival she cooled his arms with water by making him sit in the shower, as suggested by the call taker.

After ensuring that the primary survey is secure, i.e. no signs of catastrophic haemorrhage, airway patent, breathing and circulation adequate, you assess the burnt arms. Using the rule of 9s you estimate that approximately 13–15% of his body surface area (BSA) is partial-thickness burns. Robert is complaining of 7 out of 10 on the pain scale and, while making plans of how to further manage this burn and to administer a stronger type of analgesia, you let him self-administer nitrous oxide.

How long should this burn be cooled? How should the arms be dressed? What options for analgesia administration are available to you?

ANSWER & DISCUSSION

Thermal burns should be cooled with cold or tepid, running water for 20–30 minutes, as soon as possible after the injury (ideally within 20 minutes). This was already started by Robert's wife, so this should be continued until 20–30 minutes have elapsed. After cooling the burnt areas should be covered in cling film to prevent bacterial colonisation, ensuring that it is layered, rather than wrapped circumferentially to prevent vasoconstriction. Elevation is also recommended, because it can prevent oedema, which may affect healing. Now that these steps have been completed, your focus can shift to dealing with analgesia options other than nitrous oxide. Oral paracetamol, ibuprofen or paracetamol could be considered, but oral analgesics have a prolonged time until onset of action compared with intravenous drugs. However, the nitrous oxide could be the best option at this time, as intravenous access could be challenging, because both arms are injured, thus eliminating them as cannulation sites. Yes, legs could be considered as an alternative, but intravenous access might not be possible there, either. This leaves intraosseous access, but this intervention might not be available to you as Robert is conscious, and not all ambulance trusts have adopted lidocaine for intraosseous infusions in conscious patients. Your options are possibly limited to nitrous oxide administration, oral analgesics and transporting Robert in a position of comfort in a speedy fashion to allow for other drugs to be administered in the ED.

Further resources/recommended reading

National Institute for Health and Care Excellence (2017) *Burns and Scalds*, London: NICE.

PART II

MIXED CASES FOR SELF-ASSESSMENT

Christoph Schroth and Peter Phillips

CASE 21: AN ADULT MALE WITH CHEST PAIN

You have been dispatched to a private residence to a 51-year-old male with chest pain. The journey time is 6 minutes and upon arrival it is 09:15.

According to the patient's daughter, who directs you to the living room, her father developed chest pain while helping her to move into her new apartment. She got worried when he had not improved after 10 minutes, so she called an ambulance.

After introducing your colleague and yourself to the patient you begin your assessment. After your primary survey, while you are obtaining some vital signs, your colleague establishes the following history:

Allergies: None

Medication: No OTC or prescribed medication

Past medical history:

Cardiac: None

Respiratory: None

Endocrine: None

Neurological: None

Surgical: None

Occupation: English teacher

Natal: N/A

Last meal and urinary output: Breakfast was a bowl of oats and a cup of tea. Urinated about an hour ago with no abnormalities

Events leading up to the call: Was helping his daughter to move into her new apartment and developed chest pain after carrying a lot of boxes from the van into the apartment.

Examination

Alert on the AVPU scale

Equal, bilateral and clear air entry on auscultation

Strong radial pulse present (between 70 and 90 beats/minute, regular)

Not pale or diaphoretic

Vital signs

HR 90 beats/minute and regular

RR 20 breaths/minute, somewhat shallow

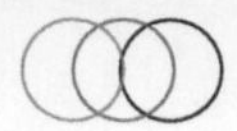

SpO_2 97% on room air

Blood pressure 140/76 mmHg

HGT 5.9 mmol/l

12-lead ECG showing normal sinus rhythm in all leads

Temperature (tympanic) 36.9°C

Pupils 4 mm, equal, round and reactive to light

What is the most likely cause of chest pain, particularly in this patient (aged >50 years), male and after some form of exercise?

What treatment and assessments are still required?

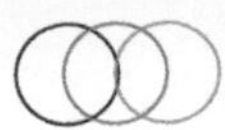

ANSWER & DISCUSSION

Chest pain due to a myocardial infarction would appear to be the most likely answer in a patient of this age, being male and aged >50 years, but does this tell the whole story? No, because this does not consider the complete picture, including the context of the onset. Looking around the apartment, it appears that most boxes are small—with the one he carried last being the biggest.

Why does this matter? Rest did not relieve the chest pain and it started after the last box was lifted. Further questioning also reveals that the pain is located in one specific area and affected by his posture. Further assessment and treatment should include a pain score and further details about its characteristics by using the OPQRST mnemonic.

Key points

- Not all chest pain is cardiac in origin.
- Vital signs, history, context, age and gender all need to be considered to reach a diagnosis.

CASE 22: PAINFUL URINATION

It is late evening and you are called to an 86-year-old female, Jennifer, who has been experiencing difficulty urinating, and her husband is concerned that she is not acting normally.

On your arrival Jennifer appears well, and engages with you as you ascertain that there are no concerns on the primary survey.

History

HPC—2-day history of a burning sensation when urinating; Jennifer has noticed that she is urinating more frequently than normal

PMH—hypertension, myocardial infarction in 2008

DHx—ramipril, aspirin, simvastatin

SHx—Jennifer lives with her husband. She is independent and enjoys a good quality of life

FHx—no significant illnesses in family

ROS—no other relevant symptoms

Vital signs

HR 88 beats/minute and regular

RR 17 breaths/minute

SpO_2 97% on room air

BP 152/93 mmHg

HGT 5.8 mmol/l

Temperature (tympanic) 38.4°C

Capillary refill time <2 seconds

GCS 15/15, although she is a little confused at times

You take a urine sample from Jennifer. The urine looks dark in colour and appears cloudy. You undertake urinalysis and are presented with the following dipstick results:

Leukocytes ++

Nitrites +

Protein negative

pH 7.6

Blood +

Ketones negative

Bilirubin negative

Glucose negative

What is your diagnosis?

Are there any symptoms/conditions that you want to rule out?

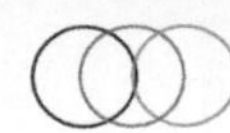

ANSWER & DISCUSSION

Jennifer is displaying the classic signs and symptoms of a lower urinary tract infection (UTI): dysuria (difficulty urinating), pyrexia and slight confusion. Traditionally, dipstick urinalysis is used to help diagnose a UTI, and Jennifer's dipstick result shows a typical UTI. However evidence suggests that the sensitivity is low, indicating that there are a large number of false-positive results. In practice, this means that urine dipsticks cannot be relied on alone to diagnose a UTI, so clinical symptoms need to form a large portion of the diagnosis. Urine dipsticks do, however, have a reasonable specificity, which means that they are useful for ruling out a UTI.

Before treating Jennifer with antibiotics for a lower UTI, you must rule out any renal involvement by ensuring that there is no kidney tenderness and no frank blood in the urine. In addition, any signs of sepsis dictate a more aggressive management plan in hospital.

Further resources/recommended reading

Health Protection Agency (2017) *Diagnosis of UTI: Quick Reference Guide for Primary Care*, London: HPA

National Institute for Health and Care Excellence (2015) *Lower Urinary Tract Infection Guidelines*, London: NICE.

CASE 23: SHORTNESS OF BREATH AT A LOCAL SCHOOL

Following an 8-minute response to a local high school, you are guided to an office in the administration building. According to the staff member showing you the way, the patient is one of their new staff members, a 28-year-old female by the name of Becky. He is not sure what exactly happened, but says that she suddenly turned pale and began breathing very fast while talking on the phone. She was breathing so fast that she could not speak properly, and he and his colleagues decided to call 999.

The primary survey, consisting of scene safety, catastrophic haemorrhage check, airway, breathing and circulation reveals only two key findings: shortness of breath without wheezing and a pale appearance. However, the patient appears to be holding her hands in an awkward position, fingertips touching the thumb, forming a curved position. Is this relevant to the case? Could this be a clue?

ANSWER & DISCUSSION

A panic attack can be triggered by a variety of events and lead to psychogenic shock, as in this case. Physical manifestations of severe psychological stress can be initially misleading, because, with every step of the assessment, the absence of specific findings does not help with narrowing down the cause of the current presentation. History and circumstances can be particularly important, such as in this case, but the hand positioning is a key clue.

Hyperventilation, as often present in episodes of severe anxiety, may trigger carpopedal spasms of the wrists and ankles, due to hypocapnia from exhaling excessive amounts of carbon dioxide as a result of the fast respiratory rate. This is often painful and a bodily response to alkalosis, because carbon dioxide levels are directly linked to cellular pH levels.

Potential signs and symptoms of anxiety attacks/panic attacks

- Hyperventilation;
- Tachycardia;
- Chest pain;
- Tremors;
- Palpitations;
- Sweating;
- Nausea;
- Dizziness.

Treatment is generally supportive and should include coaching of breathing and monitoring the patient for signs of deterioration, because, once hypocapnia reaches a certain level, the patient will experience syncope (fainting). This is due to the body attempting to reset the respiratory system to achieve normal levels of oxygen and carbon dioxide, and may therefore result in trauma from the collapse itself.

CASE 24: SEIZURES IN HOME CARE

You and your colleague are sent to a 36-year-old male with continuous seizures at a private residence. The caller is the patient's father, who is looking after his chronically ill son until another carer arrives, because his regular carer cut his hand in the early hours of this morning, and is unable to come back to work this morning, as he had to get three stitches at the ED.

On arrival the father tells you that his son suffered a severe head injury in a motorbike collision two years ago and has been suffering from seizures ever since. He has had a live-in carer for the entire time and he tells you about a 'just in case' box that they keep in the house, but he says he is not familiar with what exactly that means, because he is not the main person looking after him.

What is a 'just in case' box? What does it contain? Which drugs are you likely to administer here?

ANSWER & DISCUSSION

'Just in case' boxes contain medication that may be required for managing certain presentations where the regular, prescribed medication is not delivering adequate results. Pharmacological agents such as midazolam is likely to be present in settings where patients are under continuous care and have this prescribed for administration in case of continuous seizures and kept in this box. Administration of midazolam is covered in the 2016 and 2017 JRCALC *UK Ambulance Service Clinical Practice Guidelines*, and also commonly addressed in ambulance trust policies. This is the most likely drug that you would resort to for continuous seizures, assuming the seizures are not caused by hypoxia or hypoglycaemia, and access to the 'just in case' box is vital, because the ambulance service does not tend to issue this drug to paramedics. End-of-life care or palliative care patients may also have these boxes in place, containing medication relevant to their care. These may include analgesics (such as morphine), antiemetics (such as cyclizine or levomepromazine), drugs to manage excessive secretions (such as glycopyrronium) and, of course midazolam, to manage agitation and/or seizures.

CASE 25: ACUTE COUGH

A 32-year-old male presents at a walk-in centre with a cough that he has had for 4 days. He has no deficits on the primary survey and reports the following history:

HPC: Productive cough producing yellow sputum. He has mild pleuritic pain on inspiration. He has been feeling feverish for the last couple of days

S—pain on right side of chest

O —started 3 days ago

C—sharp in nature

R—no radiation

A—no other symptoms

T—intermittent pain

E—worse on inspiration and when coughing

S—2/10

PMH: None significant

DHx: None; not taken any analgesia

Allergies: None

SHx: Lives with wife; employed as a mechanic; does not smoke

FHx: Nothing significant

ROS: Nothing relevant

Vital signs:

RR 22 breaths/minute

HR 74 beats/minute and regular

SpO_2 97% on room air

Blood pressure 132/78 mmHg

Temperature (tympanic) 38.6°C

Capillary refill time <2 seconds

GCS 15/15

Examination

You undertake a respiratory exam. On auscultation you hear coarse crackles on the right middle lobe. All other lobes are clear. When you percuss over the right middle lobe you notice that the tone is dull compared with other lobes.

What is your preferred diagnosis of this patient?

What other tests could help you to rule in or out your preferred diagnosis?

ANSWER & DISCUSSION

This patient appears to be suffering from a chest infection, most probably pneumonia. This can be differentiated from other possible diagnoses by the presence of a purulent cough producing yellow sputum and pyrexia, although a pulmonary embolism is bound to be a differential diagnosis. Pneumonia is an infection of the alveoli that is most commonly caused by bacteria, although it can be viral and fungal. Exudate pools in the alveoli, interfering with gaseous exchange and subsequently causing an accumulation of red blood cells, fibrin and neutrophils, and leading to a solid mass called consolidation. This is distinguished from acute bronchitis, which is a viral, self-limiting infection of the bronchi and bronchioles. Acute bronchitis may cause inflammation of the bronchioles but does not cause consolidation or affect the alveoli. The distinction between a normally self-limiting acute bronchitis and bacterial pneumonia may be important when considering management options. For example, bacterial pneumonia usually requires the prescription/supply of antibiotics whereas acute bronchitis normally does not. This patient is most likely to be suffering from pneumonia because he is presenting with coarse crackles and hyporesonance, located in one lobe of the lung. These findings are caused by consolidation in the alveoli. A more in-depth respiratory exam would include the following tests.

Tactile fremitus

Laying the ulnar edge of each hand over both lungs, the paramedic asks the patient to say '99'. The vibration will be conducted more readily through solid consolidation so the vibration will be stronger over the affected lobe.

Vocal fremitus

Bronchophony—auscultating the chest while the patient says '99'. The sound will be conducted more through solid consolidation and so will be heard more clearly over the affected lobe.

Egophony—auscultating the chest while the patient says 'ee'; 'ee' will be heard as 'a' over the affected lobe, indicating consolidation. Figure 2.1 summarises the findings that compare pneumonia with acute bronchitis.

Further resources/recommended reading

National Institute for Health and Care Excellence (2014) *Pneumonia in Adults*, London: NICE.

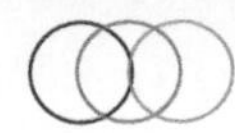

Assessment	Acute bronchitis	Community-acquired pneumonia
Cough	May or may not have sputum. Sputum less likely to be purulent	Usually have a productive cough producing yellow-, green- or rusty-coloured sputum
Auscultation	Wheeze often present, but otherwise chest clear	Coarse crackles heard over affected areas of the lungs
Percussion	Normal/resonant	Dullness/hyporesonance heard over affected areas
Vocal fremitus	Negative bronchophony and egophony	Positive bronchophony—'99' heard clearly on auscultation Positive egophony—'ee' heard as 'a' on auscultation
Tactile fremitus	Vibration equal over all areas of the lung	Increased vibration felt over affected area

Figure 2.1 Acute bronchitis versus community-acquired pneumonia

CASE 26: SINGLE VEHICLE ROLLOVER INCIDENT WITH MULTIPLE PATIENTS

During a night shift, you are driving back to station from a local hospital in a rural area when you come across a bus lying on its side next to the road. There are multiple patients walking around, people shouting for help, and pieces of luggage and debris spread across the road and the adjacent field. You position your vehicle upwind of the scene and before getting out your vehicle you declare a major incident using the mnemonic METHANE:

M (major incident declared)—Control, RRV207 declaring a major incident!

E (exact location)—High Post Corner in Salisbury

T (type of incident)—single vehicle rollover incident involving one bus

H (hazards)—no immediate threats to rescuers, but road closure essential

A (access routes)—access from both directions possible, large open space for triage and staging available next to the incident location

N (estimated number of casualties and suspected nature of injuries)—estimated 35 casualties, mostly adults with traumatic injuries from the rollover

E (emergency services)—'I am currently the only emergency service on scene, require police, fire, HART, HEMS and additional ambulances. Over.'

Now that further resources have been dispatched you exit your vehicle, grab your mass casualty kit (triage tags, glow sticks, personal protective equipment [PPE]) and head towards the bus. While walking, one question keeps on running through your mind: Can I remember the triage sieve?

Before moving on to the next page, take a blank piece of paper and draw the triage sieve from memory, if you can recall it, or make a few notes about all aspects of it that come to mind.

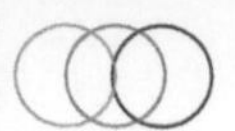

ANSWER & DISCUSSION

Mass casualty incidents (MCIs for short) are not an everyday occurrence, so the challenge is the same as treating a patient with a rare condition: trying to remember key pieces of information and putting them to good use when the time comes. The National Ambulance Resilience Unit (NARU) played a significant role in the recent revision of the triage sieve algorithm and, as with any initial patient assessment, it starts with catastrophic haemorrhage, airway and breathing, and ends with circulation (CABC). Patients are divided into four categories, priority 1 (P1), priority 2 (P2), priority 3 (P3) and priority 4 (P4—dead).

Familiarise yourself with the NARU triage sieve in Figure 2.2 and work through some imaginary examples using all possible answers at least once.

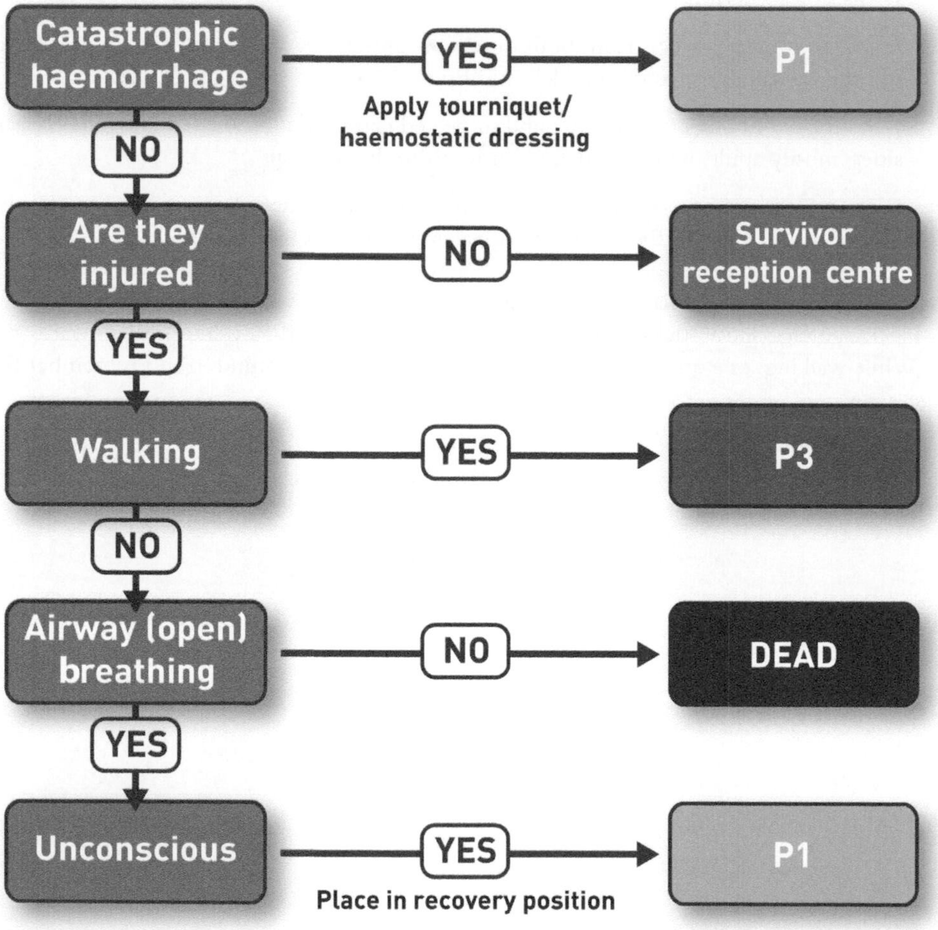

Catastrophic haemorrhage — YES → P1 (Apply tourniquet/ haemostatic dressing)

NO ↓

Are they injured — NO → Survivor reception centre

YES ↓

Walking — YES → P3

NO ↓

Airway (open) breathing — NO → DEAD

YES ↓

Unconscious — YES → P1 (Place in recovery position)

Figure 2.2 Triage sieve (reproduced with kind permission of the National Ambulance Resilience Unit (NARU))

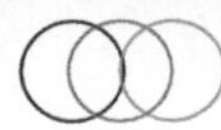

What triage priority are the following patients?

Patient A: No catastrophic haemorrhage, not injured and walking

Patient B: Catastrophic haemorrhage

Patient C: No catastrophic haemorrhage, injured, not walking and not breathing

Patient D: No catastrophic haemorrhage, injured, not walking, breathing, not unconscious, RR of 22 breaths/minute, HR of 90 beats/minute

Answers

A: Survivor reception centre;

B: P1 (apply a tourniquet or haemostatic dressing);

C: Dead;

D: P2.

CASE 27: MANAGING ASTHMA IN A 21-YEAR-OLD FEMALE

You are working on a double-crewed ambulance and are called to a 21-year-old female called Gemma who is suffering from an asthma attack. A primary survey reveals a patient who is slightly pale and diaphoretic, has a raised work of breathing using accessory muscles and is audibly wheezing.

Initial vital signs

HR 120 beats/minute

RR 30 breaths/minute

SpO_2 88% on room air

You quickly identify that Gemma is having a severe asthma attack, and that the deficits identified on the primary survey require immediate treatment. What would be a systematic way to treat Gemma? You acknowledge that undertaking a full history is not appropriate with primary survey deficits, but what information would be pertinent to collect to inform your possible treatment plan?

ANSWER & DISCUSSION

Gemma's pulse-oximetry readings are low, so the first priority is to administer oxygen. The audible wheeze indicates bronchospasm and this is the cause of low saturations, because ventilation is impaired by narrowing of the bronchioles.

Salbutamol, a β_2 agonist, should be nebulised with oxygen as soon as it is available. Oxygen should be set to between 6 and 8 litres/minute to achieve the highest quality of aerosolisation of the drug. β_2-Receptors are found predominately in the lungs and form part of the sympathetic nervous response, which relaxes smooth muscle in the bronchioles. Using salbutamol to activate β_2-receptors will help to reduce bronchospasm.

Ipratropium bromide, a cholinergic antagonist, should also be nebulised, in this case together with salbutamol. Acetylcholine is the neurotransmitter at the neuromuscular junction of the parasympathetic nervous system. Blocking the action of acetylcholine in the lungs reduces the parasympathetic response, which would cause smooth muscle contraction, in order to further relax smooth muscle and reduce bronchospasm.

The administration of corticosteroids should be considered. In this case, intravenous hydrocortisone could be administered, and indeed is recommended by JRCALC (2017). Hydrocortisone, in general, suppresses the immune system. There is an ongoing debate around the need to administer this pre-hospitally because an immediate action is unlikely; rather one would expect an improvement to be seen after around 6 hours. Nevertheless, it seems intuitive that giving it early in the treatment of acute severe asthma should improve outcomes for Gemma. There is also evidence that corticosteroids increase the sensitivity of β_2-receptors to salbutamol, causing a synergistic reaction when administered simultaneously.

Regular reassessment should take place in order to assess the impact of treatment, and to identify whether Gemma is continuing to deteriorate. End-tidal CO_2 monitoring is very useful in detecting changes during an acute asthma attack and should be used where available. It is pertinent to find out if Gemma has been admitted to hospital before, and if she has had any admissions to ITU because of asthma. This helps to give an indication of the potential seriousness of her illness, and may dictate a more aggressive treatment and/or closer monitoring.

Further resources/recommended reading

Joint Royal Colleges Ambulance Liaison Committee (2017) *UK Ambulance Services Clinical Practice Guidelines*, London: JRCALC.

British Thoracic Society (2016) *British Guideline on the Management of Asthma*, London: British Thoracic Society.

CASE 28: FEBRILE KID WITH A COUGH

You are working on an RRV and are called to an 18-month-old male at 02:00. The child's mother describes that her son has been coughing all night and has a temperature. She phoned NHS 111 who were concerned that the cough was loud and hoarse, and an ambulance was called. On arrival you undertake a primary survey, which identifies a slightly elevated respiratory rate but the child appears alert and perfused, with no signs of cyanosis. You note some intercostal recession and can also hear inspiratory stridor when the child becomes agitated, but this is not present at rest. There is no evidence of bronchospasm on auscultation and, as far as you can see, there is no swelling or redness in the oropharynx. Your assessment also reveals the following.

Vital signs

HR 140 beats/minute

RR 40 breaths/minute

SpO_2 97% on room air

Temperature (tympanic) 39°C

HGT 6.2 mmol/l

Assessment

No rash or mottling of the skin

No substernal or intercostal recession

Auscultation reveals vesicular breath sounds

The child's nappies have been wet, as normal

What is your preferred diagnosis of this child?

Does this child require admission to hospital?

What is your management of this patient?

ANSWER & DISCUSSION

This child is most likely suffering from laryngotracheobronchitis (commonly called croup). Croup is a viral infection that causes swelling and pain around the larynx, trachea and bronchi, which often affects the vocal cords and causes a characteristic 'seal-like bark' and hoarse voice. Symptoms of croup vary from mild to life threatening, with NICE suggesting that all moderate, severe and life-threatening croup should be admitted to hospital. Therefore, careful assessment is important in order to identify the severity of symptoms and to ensure correct management.

The Modified Taussig Croup Score looks at the extent of stridor and recession to indicate the severity of symptoms. This child displays stridor on exertion and intercostal recession on exertion which means he falls into the category of mild. The Modified Westley Clinical Scoring System looks at the extent of stridor, recession, air entry, cyanosis and level of consciousness. Under this scoring system the child also falls into the category of mild. NICE guidelines suggest that mild croup can be managed at home with the administration of a corticosteroid, preferably a one-off dose of dexamethasone. The parents should be advised that worsening of any symptoms should result in them calling 999, and that the symptoms should reduce rapidly after roughly 48 hours. The level of parental distress should be taken into account when making decisions about the appropriateness of non-conveyance, but a good knowledge of the illness should help to reassure parents and empower them to manage appropriately.

Further resources/recommended reading

Joint Royal Colleges Ambulance Liaison Committee (2017) *UK Ambulance Services Clinical Practice Guidelines*, London: JRCALC.

National Institute for Health and Care Excellence (2017) *Croup*, London: NICE.

British Medical Association (2017) *Croup—BMJ Best Practice*, London: BMA.

CASE 29: STABBED CHEST

During an event standby, a man walks into your medical tent on site, escorted by a police officer, saying that he has been stabbed in the chest. The police officer wanted the patient to be collected by the medical team on site, but the patient insisted on walking to the medical tent. Before assessment starts the question of scene safety, i.e. the whereabouts of the suspect, needs to be answered. Luckily, the suspect has already been detained.

Instead of treating and assessing the patient in your medical tent, you choose to assess him inside your ambulance which you have standing by for transportation, because you are certain (due to the type and mechanism of injury) that a hospital assessment is urgently required. The patient is 34 years old, fully alert and orientated, and complaining of pain around the injury site on the right side of his chest. The SpO_2 on room air is at 93% and equal, bilateral air entry is present on auscultation. Respiratory rate is 18 breaths/minute and the radial pulse is palpable at a regular rate of 90 beats/minute.

The following questions need to be considered before or while en route to hospital:

Which treatment might this patient require in the very near future?

What equipment do you require?

En route you contact your chosen hospital and log a pre-alert following the ATMIST mnemonic:

A (age)—34 year-old male

T (time)—he was stabbed approximately 10 minutes ago, ETA to the hospital of about 8 minutes.

M (mechanism)—stabbed once into the right side of his chest

I (injuries)—a single, sucking chest wound between ribs 3 and 4

S (signs and symptoms)—pain at the site of injury, but no shortness of breath present or signs of significant blood loss found

T (treatment)—patient currently receiving oxygen, has a non-occlusive chest seal *in situ* and is being monitored. No other treatment undertaken yet

ANSWER & DISCUSSION

Scene safety is undoubtedly a continuous priority, but the suspect has already been detained. Catastrophic haemorrhage was not present, oxygen and a non-occlusive (vented) chest seal has been applied. These are all vital in treating a patient with a (sucking) chest wound. Despite no other significant abnormalities having been detected so far, there should be a high index of suspicion for a tension pneumothorax. A tension pneumothorax develops when the pleura around the lungs and lining the chest wall have been penetrated, allowing air to enter the pleural space, but, due to the way the tissue has aligned itself, the air cannot escape, thus creating an area of high air pressure. The resultant force limits expansion of the lung on the affected side, resulting in shortness of breath, decreased air entry, hypoxia and, if not treated, death.

A needle thoracentesis (also called needle thoracocentesis) should be undertaken if a particular set of criteria are met, such as dyspnoea, decreased air entry on the affected side, hyper-resonance on percussion, jugular venous distension (JVD) and tracheal deviation towards the unaffected side. However, JVD and tracheal deviation are late signs and not all signs and symptoms have to be present to warrant treatment. Typically, a 14G intravenous cannula or a specialised device is inserted into the second intercostal space at the mid-clavicular line or in the fifth intercostal space at the mid-axillary line to 'decompress the chest', thus allowing the lung to fully re-expand and resolve most or all symptoms.

CASE 30: FEVER IN THE RETURNING TRAVELLER

A 42-year-old male presents to the GP surgery you are working at today, complaining of flu-like symptoms: fever, lethargy, hot and cold flushes, and a headache. He says that he has been feeling unwell since returning from a 14-day work trip 2 days ago and that he took a temperature of 38.8°C at home. He has also been having hot and cold flushes, but only on the first day back and today, but has been feeling lethargic and nauseous all the time.

Some additional findings from the vital signs assessment and history are as follows:

HR 85 breaths/minute

RR 20 breaths/minute

SpO_2 of 97% on room air

BP 130/75 mmHg

Temperature (tympanic) 38.9°C

Allergies: None

Medication: Malarone® once a day for about the last 18 or 19 days, he is not sure

Past medical history: Appendectomy in 2010, but no other history of note.

Last meal: Small breakfast this morning, but nausea has reduced his appetite.

Events: Returned from a work trip to Cameroon, but has been feeling unwell ever since

Which conditions are you considering at this point?

Which reference literature could you consult to form a strong diagnosis?

ANSWER & DISCUSSION

Flu-like symptoms are a common presentation in the primary healthcare setting and are also a very generic set of symptoms that can be present in multiple conditions. To narrow down the diagnosis, focus on the key pieces that could provide you with avenues to explore. First, what is Malarone® and what is it used for? Atovaquone with proguanil hydrochloride, which the patient has been taking for a few weeks, is the generic name for Malarone®, a malaria prophylaxis medication. Second, the patient returned from Cameroon, but is that a malaria endemic region? Yes, it is a high-risk area and this information can be found in the *British National Formulary* (BNF), a publication you were probably already utilising to look up Malarone and its indications.

Based on these findings, it is highly likely that this patient is suffering from malaria, specifically a variant called falciparum malaria. This is the most dangerous variant and, as he has just returned from an endemic area, has been showing signs and symptoms of malaria, and is taking malaria prophylaxis, this is the most likely diagnosis. Other key pieces of information are the hot and cold flushes that are about 2 days apart; these are typical in falciparum malaria and called paroxysms. Fever in the returning traveller is always a concern, but even more so if they have been abroad, particularly in a subtropical region where malaria and other infectious diseases are a common occurrence. This patient requires urgent treatment and a specialist consultation to allow for the best course of treatment to be selected.

Further resources/recommended reading

British National Formulary (in print, via the smartphone app or via www.medicinescomplete.com).

CASE 31: CHILD WITH SEIZURES

You and your colleague are called at 10am to a 2-year-old male who is fitting. When you arrive on scene the child is no longer fitting but is quite drowsy, in the post-ictal phase. The mother reports that her son has had a fever for the last 24 hours, along with a dry cough and a sore throat. She was getting him ready to go to nursery for the day when his eyes 'glazed over', his body went stiff and he started shaking. The mother is unsure exactly how long it lasted but she thinks it was about 3 minutes before he stopped shaking. This has not happened before and the mother is worried that it is the start of epilepsy. You take the following vital signs:

HR 140 beats/minute

RR 25 breaths/minute

SpO_2 97% on room air

Temperature (tympanic) 38.7°C

HGT 5.6 mmol/l

After around 15 minutes the child returns to his normal level of consciousness and, although tired, the mother reports that he is much more like his normal self. At this point you consider that the child has suffered a febrile convulsion. This conclusion is well founded because the child has a feverish illness, seemed to have a tonic–clonic seizure lasting up to 3 minutes, and has recovered quickly and fully. Febrile convulsions affect children up to the age of about 5, and affect slightly more males than females.

What else do you need to consider with this patient?

Does the child require hospitalisation or further investigation?

ANSWER & DISCUSSION

A febrile convulsion occurs as a symptom of a feverish illness, most commonly a viral illness, although the pathophysiology of how this causes a seizure is not well known. The simple febrile convulsion that this child has experienced is of little concern in itself, because it was short-lasting and the recovery was quick and complete. Assessment and decision-making now need to focus on the cause of the illness, with particular attention given to ruling out meningitis, encephalitis or other focal abnormal neurology. It is often difficult to definitively rule out such illnesses in infants, so it is important that you identify the source of the infection. This requires an examination of body systems and a good history. Some common sources of infections in paediatrics are:

- Ear infections;
- Throat infections;
- Chest infections;
- Skin infections;
- Urinary tract infections.

The mother in this case has reported that her son has had a sore throat and a dry cough. It would be prudent to visualise the oropharynx and larynx to see if there is any swelling, reddening or exudate that would indicate an infection or tonsillitis. If the source of the infection cannot be found then hospital admission may be appropriate.

NICE guidelines recommend that a child suffering a first febrile convulsion be admitted to hospital for paediatric assessment. However, a simple, uncomplicated, febrile convulsion in which the source of the infection is identified could be considered low risk and could be suitable to manage at home, even if this is a first occurrence. This is particularly true for children over 18 months old, although you may have a lower threshold for admitting to hospital in younger infants.

In this case, a throat infection seems to be the source of the infection, which is usually viral and self-limiting. This child could safely be left in the care of his mother with advice to call 999 again should symptoms worsen or should the child have another convulsion. The mother should be reassured that this type of seizure does not cause long-term damage and is not correlated with the risk of developing epilepsy.

Further resources/recommended reading

National Institute for Health and Care Excellence (2013) *Febrile Seizure*, London: NICE
National Institute for Health and Care Excellence (2017) *Fever in Under 5s*, London: NICE
Spotting the sick child: https://www.spottingthesickchild.com

CASE 32: COLLAPSED MAN IN THE PARK

An unresponsive man is found by a police patrol in a local park and an ambulance arrives on scene within minutes. You are the senior officer on shift and decide to stop by with your response vehicle to see if your colleagues need any assistance.

Alcohol intoxication is a frequent reason for calls to the police and the ambulance service, and patients often turn out to be intoxicated, rather than medically unwell, but this still means that it needs to be investigated and that any serious causes of collapse are ruled out. Depending on the time of the year, hypothermia is also a major concern, particularly when alcohol intoxication is suspected, but what else causes unresponsiveness or depresses the central nervous or cardiovascular system?

Here are some to consider:

- Alcohol;
- Hypothermia;
- Cerebrovascular accident (CVA) or transient ischaemic attack (TIA);
- Hypoglycaemia;
- Seizures (absence seizures or the post-ictal phase);
- Hypoxia.

What are some other causes you could consider?

ANSWER & DISCUSSION

Causes of unconsciousness are numerous and not all can be completely assessed in the pre-hospital setting. One mnemonic often taught in emergency care courses is AEIOUTIPS, which provides a framework to guide you towards the potential causes:

A—alcohol

E—endocrine and electrolytes

I—insulin

O—opiates and oxygen deficiency (hypoxia)

U—uraemia (renal problems)

T—trauma (head injury, haemorrhagic shock) and temperature

I—intracranial pressure and infection

P—poisoning and psychiatric causes

S—seizures, sepsis, stroke, shock and syncope

CASE 33: PATIENT WITH CLOTTING PROBLEMS

You have been dispatched to a local assisted-living facility; despite this call requiring a specialist paramedic to attend, you are the only available vehicle and the call has been pending for quite a while. The dispatch information you were given stated only: 'Clotting disorder, patient requires advice. Specialist paramedic not available at this time.'

The patient is a 78-year-old male with dementia; a family member welcomes you and explains that they are concerned after having read all their father's medical paperwork from the GP and that something 'is just not right with his blood work'. Before exploring these concerns in more detail, you introduce yourself to the patient, Robert Johnson, and undertake a primary survey to ensure that no immediately life-threatening problems require any urgent attention. The primary survey is secure and now you explore the concerns of the family. Before you even manage to read through the notes, she hands you a piece of paper with a laboratory report she found in Robert's medical file from his GP dated last week (see below):

Patient: Robert Johnson (male, 78 years old)

Haemoglobin: 14.7 g/dl (reference value 13.0–18.0 mg/dl)

Blood glucose: 5.7 mmol/l (reference value 3.5–7.0 mmol/l for non-fasting glucose)

INR 3.8 (reference value 0.9–1.2)

PT 19 seconds (reference value 12.7–15.0 seconds)

The results are not something you deal with all the time and, even if you called the clinical help desk, you would need to know what you should be asking them about. Which of these figures are of concern to you?

Which element of the history do you need to ask particular questions about, in order to make the most of the laboratory report?

ANSWER & DISCUSSION

Blood tests normally have reference values printed next to the current results, thus allowing healthcare providers to easily identify potential clues towards making a diagnosis. Prothrombin time (PT) and international normalised ratio (INR) are two key terms when dealing with patients with clotting disorders, but these cannot be accurately evaluated or commented on, without knowing which medication the patient is currently taking. Warfarin, a platelet aggregation inhibitor, is the key drug here, because the INR is the value of interest in patients on anticoagulation therapy, although the PT is important for all other patients. Hence, confirming the medication that Robert is currently taking is important.

A call to the clinical support desk, the patient's GP or specialist, if he currently is under the care of one, would enable you to make a more informed, patient-centred decision. Options may include: hospital admission, arranging a review or appointment, or attempting to request a specialist paramedic to come around again, if your scope of practice does not allow for a suitable intervention to be performed at this time.

CASE 34: SHORTNESS OF BREATH

When assessing a 62-year-old female who is short of breath at a private home you discover pulmonary oedema in both lower lobes while auscultating, but no wheeze. The reason for the call to 999 was for shortness of breath that became progressively worse over the last 5–7 days. During the assessment you notice a packet of tablets on the bedside table that is part of the thiazide family and, according to the patient, she takes half a tablet a day for her shortness of breath. Further history taking reveals that she suffers from congestive cardiac failure and that she picked up her new prescription about a week ago, because her previous supply of tablets had come to an end. Looking at the label on the new medication packet you notice that it says: 'Take 1–2 tablets per day'; however, the patient said she takes ½ a tablet per day. Could this be the cause of the worsening pulmonary oedema, i.e. under-dosing?

ANSWER & DISCUSSION

Congestive cardiac failure is clearly the diagnosis here, which became evident due to a thorough history and paying attention to the environmental clues (i.e. the medication packet and a potential dosage error). Without this, it would have been significantly more difficult to establish what was causing the pulmonary oedema. Unfortunately, the old medication packets are not available to compare the label, but a phone call to her doctor confirms your suspicions; he prescribed one to two tablets per day. Human error, not a change in the patient's condition, is the most likely cause of the worsening shortness of breath here, but hospital evaluation might still be justified, depending on the feedback from her doctor. Pulmonary oedema itself is not a diagnosis, but a symptom of an underlying condition or event. Treatment with loop diuretics, such as furosemide, or thiazide class diuretics, such as hydrochlorothiazide, is often already under way when the ambulance service gets called to such scenarios as this case. Most guidelines recommend the use of GTN (glyceryl trinitrate) sublingual spray as the first-line treatment for acute pulmonary oedema secondary to congestive cardiac failure, and it generally provides quick relief; it does, however, not address the underlying cause of the pulmonary oedema or help with identifying the cause. In this case, the onset is not acute, raising the question of whether GTN should be used. Depending on the severity of the respiratory distress and it being secondary to congestive cardiac failure, GTN should definitely be considered, because it meets the criteria of most clinical guidelines, but investigations to find the actual cause should continue.

Further resources/recommended reading

British National Formulary (in print, via the smartphone app or via www.medicinescomplete.com).

CASE 35: END-OF-LIFE CANCER CARE

It is 03:00 and you are working for the GP out-of-hours service and are called to a palliative care patient who is becoming increasingly breathless. The patient is a 59-year-old female who has ovarian cancer with bone metastases, and is being treated palliatively. The family inform you that she is having no more chemotherapy, she does not want active treatment, and the focus is now on making her comfortable so she can die at home. Over the last week the patient has become increasingly weak and tired, and is now virtually bed-bound. The family report that the patient has been getting increasingly breathless over the last 24 hours, and she is now becoming quite agitated. Auscultation reveals vesicular breath sounds, no signs of secretions and no obvious cause of dyspnoea. You note that there are just-in-case medications along with a drugs chart, and that none of the medication has yet been given.

What is this patient's prognosis?

What options should you consider for managing this situation?

ANSWER & DISCUSSION

You may find documentation (such as treatment escalation plans, ceiling of treatment plans or similar documents) that would give an indication of the patient's prognosis. However, this patient is displaying signs that she is rapidly deteriorating and may be entering her last days of life. In the last days of life it is not uncommon for patients to become breathless. Breathlessness could be caused by a myriad of aetiologies in the terminal phase, but simple measures can be used in all cases to try to relieve symptoms.

The patient should be reassured that this feeling of breathlessness can be reduced and that you will help her. She should be sat up as much as is possible, and a fan (or open window) can be used to blow air over the patient's face, which reduces the feeling of breathlessness. Opioids are effective at reducing the perception of breathlessness and, where governance permits, oral or subcutaneous morphine can be administered in small doses. There is little value in taking any vital signs because you are not likely to act on any abnormal findings.

Reducing the feeling of breathlessness may also reduce the level of agitation. Agitation is another common symptom at the end of life and a benzodiazepine can be effective at reducing it. Therefore, if agitation does not reduce then a benzodiazepine, such as midazolam, can be used and should be found with the just-in-case medication. It is important to record your assessment and interventions in the patient's notes, and to inform the patient's GP or palliative care team of your visit to ensure continuation of care. It is prudent to note that her palliative care team may not be aware of her deterioration this week so she may need an urgent review.

Further resources/recommended reading

National Institute for Health and Care Excellence (2016) *Palliative Care: Dyspnoea*, London: NICE.
National Institute for Health and Care Excellence (2016) *Palliative Care: General issues*, London: NICE.
The Gold Standards Framework: www.goldstandardsframework.org.uk.

CASE 36: PATIENT ON A VENTILATOR

During an ambulance shift you are scheduled to conduct an inter-hospital transfer of an intubated and ventilated adult male patient together with a nurse and a doctor, who will be escorting the patient. Although it is not your responsibility to manage this patient independently, you may be called on to assist. During your wait for the patient to be made ready for transport, you carefully study the dials, buttons and settings of the ventilator. Some of the terms and abbreviations you encounter are:

VT, RR, MV, I:E, FiO_2, Peak flow and CMV.

Are you familiar with these terms, abbreviations, associated calculations and recommended settings?

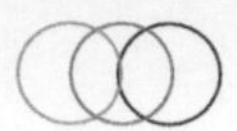

ANSWER & DISCUSSION

VT stands for tidal volume and is often written as V_T, which can be calculated by multiplying the patients weight in kilograms by 5–7 ml/kg (*V*T = kg × 5–7 ml or *V*T = 5–7 ml/kg).

RR stands for respiratory rate and is normally the rate the patient is breathing at, but in the case of a ventilated patient it refers to the rate pre-set for the patient; 8–10 breaths/minute is the typical range for intubated patients, but this may be adjusted depending on $ETCO_2$ levels and other factors.

MV stands for minute volume, which is calculated by multiplying respiratory rate by the tidal volume, giving you a minute volume in millilitres (MV = RR × *V*T).

I:E stands for inspiratory to expiratory ratio and is typically 1:2. In other words, for every second it takes to breathe in, it takes 2 seconds to breathe out, or breathing out takes twice as long as breathing in.

FiO_2 stands for fraction of inspired oxygen and is expressed in values between 0 and 1. For example, FiO_2 of 0.3 equals 30% of inspired oxygen, whereas FiO_2 of 1 equals 100% oxygen. Setting the FiO_2 to 0 would imply that no oxygen supplementation is taking place and that the patient is breathing only room air.

Peak flow refers to the speed at which the set tidal volume (*V*T) is delivered, i.e. how fast each ventilation is delivered.

CMV stands for continuous manual ventilation and ensures that the ventilator delivers a set volume and rate of breaths every minute, regardless of the patient's respiratory effort. This mode is mostly used in apnoeic or sedated patients.

For this patient VT and MV would be calculated using these two formulas (examples of calculations below):

$$VT = 5\text{–}7 \text{ ml/kg} = 380\text{–}532 \text{ ml/minute}$$

(With 5 ml/kg = 76 kg × 5 ml = 380 ml; with 6 ml/kg = 76 kg × 6 ml = 456 ml; and with 7 ml/kg = 76 kg × 7 ml = 532 ml)

$$MV = RR \times VT$$

At a respiratory rate of 8 breaths/minute and 380 ml of tidal volume:

$$MV = 8 \text{ breaths/minute} \times 380 \text{ ml} = 3040 \text{ ml}.$$

In case the ventilator should fail you need to ensure that you have a bag–valve–mask (BVM) on hand to ventilate the patient, and a suction unit nearby to allow you to clear secretions from the airway.

CASE 37: ANKLE INJURY

You are working in a minor injuries unit on a Saturday and are presented with a 25-year-old male who has sustained an ankle injury. You watch him hobble from the waiting room into the treatment room and can see that he is in pain, but is able to put some weight on his right foot. You take the following focused history:

HPC: He was playing football when he was tackled and inverted his right ankle which caused him to fall over

S—pain on right-hand side of ankle

O—after being tackled

C—sharp pain

R—no radiation

A—none

T—constant pain

E—worse on palpation of right malleolus

S—4/10

PMH: None significant

DHx: None; not taken any analgesia

Allergies: None

SHx: Lives alone; works as an IT technician

FHx: Nothing relevant

ROS: No other injuries

How would you assess this patient to determine if an X-ray is appropriate?

ANSWER & DISCUSSION

The Ottawa foot and ankle rules were designed to try to reduce the number of unnecessary X-rays where there is a clear history of twisting of the ankle.

In accordance with the Ottawa rules, you first need to ascertain whether the patient is able to weight bear on his right foot for four steps, but you have already observed this when he was walking into the treatment room, so an X-ray is not indicated on these grounds.

Pain over the tip of either malleolus or pain up the posterior edge of the tibia/fibula is an indication for an X-ray. Therefore, you need to palpate over these areas to ascertain if the pain is specifically over the bone or isolated to the ligaments that run below the malleolus. It can often be difficult to distinguish malleolar pain from ligament damage, so careful and precise palpation is needed.

The foot criteria of the Ottawa rules dictate that an X-ray is undertaken if there is pain over the navicular bone or at the base of the fifth metatarsal. Therefore, it is important to precisely palpate these bones which requires a good knowledge of the anatomy of the foot. You find that there is pain isolated to the lateral malleolus, which, according to the Ottawa rules, indicates that an X-ray needs to be undertaken.

Further resources/recommended reading

National Institute for Health and Care Excellence (2016) *Sprains and Strains*, London: NICE.

Stiell, I., Wells, G., Laupacis, A. et al. (1995) Multicentre trial to introduce the Ottawa ankle rules for use of radiography in acute ankle injuries, *British Medical Journal*, 311, 594

CASE 38: INJURY FROM AN AXE

A 34-year-old male called the ambulance service after injuring his leg with an axe this morning. He used his T-shirt as a dressing and applied direct pressure, but it kept on bleeding, so he dialled 999. On your arrival in a rapid response vehicle an ambulance crew is already on scene and has applied a tourniquet to the left leg.

After speaking to the patient it becomes apparent how this injury occurred. He was attempting to chop some tree roots in his garden, but the axe bounced off and hit the left lateral aspect of the tibia/fibula, leaving a large laceration.

According to your evaluation of the wound, you think it could be managed without a tourniquet. Wound packing is your preferred option, but can you safely remove a tourniquet, once applied? What are the key considerations here? What methods might you have to employ to manage the bleeding?

ANSWER & DISCUSSION

Initial application of a tourniquet to what appears to be an exsanguinating haemorrhage is vital, but sometimes the initial presentation is different from the actual extent of the injury. In such cases, removal of a tourniquet may be warranted, but has to meet certain criteria before this can be done. In pre-hospital care the removal of an arterial tourniquet is not often necessary, but, due to the widespread availability of these devices, the situation will come when this has to be considered. Tourniquets can generally be left in place for approximately 2 hours without any long-term complications, but the timeframe for safe removal after application, where the decision was made to pack the wound and/or apply a pressure dressing to manage the bleeding, is not clearly defined. In some literature and ambulance trust guidelines a 30-minute time limit is mentioned, but the origin of this timeframe is not entirely clear. However, removal of a tourniquet beyond a reasonable timeframe, such as the 30-minute one, for example, may have detrimental consequences, because the accumulation of potassium from ischaemic muscles and tissues may lead to dysrhythmias and cardiac arrest, due to the sudden influx into the circulatory system on removal of the tourniquet. Please use your catastrophic haemorrhage guidelines to identify the applicable algorithm in your area of work. Other treatment considerations include the choice of wound packing material, i.e. haemostatic agent versus untreated gauze, the potential need to cannulate and the decision whether tranexamic acid should be considered.

The type of wound packing material may be largely up to the equipment you have available, and your professional opinion of the severity of bleeding to decide between a haemostatic agent and untreated gauze. Administration of tranexamic acid is contraindicated if the bleeding has already stopped, as in this case.

CASE 39: REFUSAL OF CARE

You are first on scene of a patient who was reported as having fallen in the town centre. On arrival you are presented with a female patient in her mid-50s surrounded by numerous bystanders, sitting on a park bench. You are welcomed by one of the bystanders before you can even introduce yourself to the patient, who explains that she saw the patient trip and fall on the pavement, and that she needs to be 'given a once over by the paramedics' because she could have hurt herself. After introducing yourself to the patient, she immediately tells you that she is fine and needs no help and does not want to be assessed. You notice no obvious signs of injury, and no blood on her clothes or on the pavement. The bystanders apparently called the ambulance, even though she did not want them to.

Do you require a signed refusal of care form to depart the scene? What about the insistent bystander(s): could they be giving you a clue towards potentially invisible injuries? Could her insistence to refuse medical care be a sign of a medical condition or is she merely annoyed by the bystander's insistence to get her an ambulance?

ANSWER & DISCUSSION

Refusal of care is nothing unusual and when the patient did not call the ambulance herself, but was pushed towards waiting for the paramedics to arrive, 'just in case something is wrong', this can lead to somewhat stressful interactions between all involved parties.

Differential diagnoses for this patient could include numerous possibilities: Concussion (due to the potential fall), CVA/TIA (due to the patient's age), hypoglycaemia or soft-tissue injuries. The question is, however, whether these are valid or if the reason the patient is refusing care is because she is actually fine. The bystanders could have over-reacted and this led to a tense situation. Resolving this situation is not easy and the option that this patient has a serious medical condition does exist, but, in order to manage this scene effectively, a few key points should be considered/addressed:

- Observe patient and bystander behaviour;
- Evaluate the scene of the incident for potential clues about the mechanism of injury;
- Discuss the events with the caller/bystanders;
- Attempt to explain to the patient why you are here and that you have only her wellbeing in mind;
- Document everything you see, hear and consider in as much detail as possible

CASE 40: EPISTAXIS

You are called to a 78-year-old male who is suffering from a nosebleed (epistaxis). On arrival at his house you see that his chin and the front of his shirt are covered in blood. You undertake a primary survey and find no deficits, although he is finding it difficult to breathe through his nose and keeps spitting out blood, so you decide that stopping the bleeding is a priority to prevent potential airway issues.

Do you know the appropriate simple first aid measures to control epistaxis?

You effectively stop the bleeding, which you noticed was coming out of the right nostril, and take a set of vital signs and a history:

HR 84 beats/minute and irregular

RR 16 breaths/minute

BP 176/86 mmHg

SpO_2 97% on room air

Temperature (tympanic) 36.6°C

History

HPC: Epistaxis started spontaneously 1 hour ago, the patient has had his head tipped back but has been unable to stop the bleeding. This has not happened before

PMH: Hypertension, atrial fibrillation

DHx: Ramipril, simvastatin, warfarin

Allergies: None

SHx: Lives with his wife; both are independent

FHx: Nothing relevant

ROS: Nothing relevant

What is a likely cause of this epistaxis?

What would be an appropriate management plan?

ANSWER & DISCUSSION

Epistaxis can be categorised by whether the site of bleeding is in the posterior or the anterior portion of the nose. A posterior epistaxis will often present with blood coming out of both nostrils, and/or blood going into the oropharynx. An anterior epistaxis will usually present with blood coming out of one nostril only, and will generally result in less blood loss.

This patient is presenting with an anterior epistaxis where simple first aid measures may be sufficient to stop bleeding. The patient should lean his head forward and the soft part of the nose should be pinched for 10–15 minutes without letting go. The application of an icepack to the nose has no proven benefit. The cause of the epistaxis should be considered because this is likely to inform the management plan. This patient is taking a common anticoagulant, warfarin, which will increase blood loss and may make the epistaxis more difficult to terminate. You should check his last INR results, which will be recorded in his yellow anticoagulant book, to ensure that it is within the desired range, and refer any concerns to the GP. Once the epistaxis has been terminated, then the patient may be safe to be discharged at home. He should be advised not to blow his nose, not to lie flat, and not to drink hot drinks or alcohol for 24 hours.

You should have a lower threshold for admission if you are unable to stop the bleeding, if there is significant blood loss or there is a concerning underlying cause for the epistaxis.

Further resources/recommended reading

National Institute for Health and Care Excellence (2015) *Epistaxis*, London: NICE.

CASE 41: 'DO I START RESUSCITATION?'

You are working on an ambulance and are called to an elderly female patient who has activated her careline alarm but staff cannot make voice contact with her. On arrival the police have already forced entry into the house because they saw the elderly female lying unconscious in her bedroom. In addition, the patient's daughter has arrived because careline contacted her. The police have started chest compressions and state that they had done so within 9 minutes of the careline being activated. The patient's daughter informs you that the patient has a 'Do Not Attempt Resuscitation (DNAR)' order in place and presents you with a photocopy. You have some concerns about the validity of the DNAR but need to make a decision on whether to attempt resuscitation. Your concerns are:

- It is a photocopy. Do I need to see the original?
- There is no expiry date on the DNAR.
- The patient is not aware of the DNAR.
- Does the DNAR cover the cause of this cardiac arrest?

ANSWER & DISCUSSION

Decisions about not starting or ceasing resuscitation attempts are emotive and carry significant responsibility. The presence of a DNAR indicates that medical professionals involved in the patient's care have concluded that, in the event of cardiac arrest, resuscitation attempts would not be in the patient's best interests. Ideally the patient will have been involved in the decision-making process; however, this may not always be possible and does not invalidate a DNAR if it has not been done.

It is good practice for DNARs to be reviewed as the condition of the patient changes. However, there is no requirement to have an expiry date on a DNAR.

It is not best practice to have photocopies of DNARs, because if it is subsequently retracted or altered then it may not be possible to keep track of photocopies. However, it is reasonable to assume that the photocopy of this DNAR is valid unless there is clear evidence to the contrary.

If there are exceptions to enacting the DNAR, for example if the event leading to cardiac arrest does not amount to a natural end of life, is easily reversible or was not the circumstances envisaged when the DNAR decision was made, it may be appropriate to start resuscitation. However, these events are extremely rare.

DNARs should guide the clinician on resuscitation decisions. You should use them in the spirit that they are intended—that a healthcare professional who knows the patient well (and possibly the patient him- or herself) has concluded that a resuscitation attempt would not be in the best interests of the patient in most circumstances.

Further resources/recommended reading

British Medical Association, Resuscitation Council (UK) and Royal College of Nursing (2016) *Decisions Relating to Cardiopulmonary Resuscitation*, 3rd edition, London: BMA.
General Medical Council, *Cardiopulmonary Resuscitation*, London: General Medical Council.
Resuscitation Council (UK) *Do Not Attempt CPR*, London: Resuscitation Council (UK).

CASE 42: CHEST PAIN AND HYPOTENSION

A 48-year-old male with retrosternal chest pain, who is pale and diaphoretic, is being treated for an anteroseptal ST-elevation myocardial infarction (STEMI). The medical history reveals no allergies and a previous acute myocardial infarction in 2014, for which he had two stents inserted. Regular medication is only aspirin, once a day. His wife confirms that he presented the same way when he had his last heart attack, so she knew that an ambulance was urgently required. His blood pressure is assessed before administering two puffs of sublingual glyceryl trinitrate spray (GTN), 135/75 mmHg. Shortly after the GTN is administered the patient is complaining of severe dizziness and light-headedness. A second BP is obtained of 70/40 mmHg.

Why is his blood pressure this low? What are the potential causes of this significant drop?

ANSWER & DISCUSSION

Hypotension can lead to dizziness and confusion, but this significant drop in this patient's BP is not a typical result of GTN administration, suggesting that there are other contributing factors present. Contraindications for the administration of GTN include: hypotension, hypovolaemia, head injury and sildenafil use in the last 24 hours. The simple oversight of asking about the use of Viagra® (sildenafil) or similar drugs in the last 24 hours is the most likely cause here. Yes, sildenafil is generally contraindicated in cardiac patients, but a large percentage of erectile dysfunction medication is not obtained via the official routes (GP or specialist), but via overseas, mail order from online retailers. Second, the presence of the patient's wife in the room during the medical history assessment is not likely to motivate the patient to disclose such personal information, because erectile dysfunction is often not openly discussed, even with long-term partners. From 2018 Viagra® (sildenafil) is available as an over-the-counter medication from pharmacies in the UK, which should address the issues around overseas procurement of pharmaceuticals that are often of low-grade quality.

CASE 43: INGESTION OF LAUNDRY DETERGENT

You and your colleague are called to attend to a 14-year-old male who apparently ingested laundry detergent. His mother called 999 after finding a video on her son's social media page showing him placing some of her laundry detergent pods in his mouth and bursting them. Apparently this is known as 'tide popping', he told her on being confronted. She meets you at the door and leads you to Alan's room. Alan immediately interacts with you, asking you if he is trouble and if you are going to have to take him to hospital. You introduce yourself and your colleague and explain that you will have to undertake some assessments and then you will make some decisions, together with him and his mother, about the need to go to hospital.

His primary survey and vital signs reveal no abnormalities, with only a slight smell of laundry detergent from his airway giving a clue that he had been exposed to some kind of laundry detergent.

Does Alan need to go to hospital? What other actions might you have to take?

ANSWER & DISCUSSION

The activity of placing laundry detergent pods in one's mouth and popping them, all while filming this and posting it on social media afterwards, is known as tide popping. This is not a completely new trend, but does carry significant toxicological risks due to its combination of ingredients. Does this mean that this is going to become a major trend in the developed world? No, because the number of reported cases of 'tide popping', which got its name from an American product of a similar name, is fairly low. But it highlights the potential challenges that keep on evolving in the pre-hospital care sector, thus making it paramount that you are aware where to find further information. Your options could include: calling the clinical support desk, speaking to ED, consulting Toxbase.org via the app or a computer, or contacting area-specific toxicology support services. Hospitalisation is not likely to be required, but the above-mentioned services should be consulted to aid in your decision-making process. A safeguarding referral may also be indicated.

CASE 44: PALPITATIONS

You and your colleague are called to a 32-year-old female who is experiencing palpitations and feels like her 'heart is racing'. On arrival at her house you see that she is sitting on her sofa, looks slightly pale and states that she feels a little light-headed. She does not have chest pain and has never experienced anything like this before. You take her vital signs:

HR 190 beats/minute and regular, radial pulse present

RR 16 breaths/minute

BP 103/65 mmHg

SpO_2 98% on room air

You conduct a 12-lead ECG, which shows a narrow QRS complex with a regular rhythm at 190 beats/minute.

Which diagnosis do you consider most likely?

What would be an appropriate management plan?

ANSWER & DISCUSSION

This patient is suffering from a narrow complex tachycardia, also known a supraventricular tachycardia (SVT). The QRS complexes are narrow because the impulse originates from above the ventricles; in this case the impulse is most likely to be originating in the sinoatrial (SA) node.

The rhythm is regular, which means that it is unlikely to be fast atrial fibrillation, which would necessitate conveyance to an ED. Instead vagal manoeuvres should be attempted in order to terminate the tachycardia, which should also terminate the symptoms of palpitations and light-headedness. Vagal manoeuvres stimulate the vagus nerve, which has a parasympathetic effect on the heart, thus slowing the heart rate down. There are numerous vagal manoeuvres that you can try. The modified Valsalva manoeuvre has been shown to have a greater success rate than the traditional Valsalva manoeuvre with very little side effects, provided that her blood pressure is >90 mmHg systolic. This is achieved by having the patient in a semi-recumbent position and asking her to blow through either a tube connected to a blood pressure cuff gauge (to achieve a pressure of 40 mmHg) or a syringe so the plunger moves for 15 seconds. Immediately lie the patient down with her straight legs raised at 45° for 15 seconds and return them to the semi-recumbent position. Once the SVT has been terminated you should check for signs of atrioventricular (AV) re-entrant tachycardias, which are characterised by a short P–R interval and, in the case of Wolff–Parkinson–White syndrome, a delta wave. If these signs are present, then a referral to cardiology would be warranted. If the rhythm returns to a normal sinus rhythm, then it would be safe to assume that the cause of the SVT was an AV node re-entrant tachycardia, which does not require follow-up unless further problems occur. If vagal manoeuvres do not terminate the SVT, then chemical cardioversion is likely to be required in an ED, with adenosine usually being the first-line anti-arrhythmic drug for this type of SVT.

Further resources/recommended reading

Resuscitation Council (UK) *Adult Tachycardia (with pulse) Algorithm*, London: Resuscitation Council (UK).

The REVERT Trial, *A Modified Valsalva Maneuver to Convert SVT*, available at: http://rebelem.com/the-revert-trial-a-modified-valsalva-maneuver-to-convert-svt.

CASE 45: SMOKE INHALATION

A waiter at a local restaurant discovered a fire in a storeroom and managed to extinguish it with a fire extinguisher. He is now coughing and short of breath, but fully alert and orientated. The CFR (community first responder) who arrived before you is already administering oxygen via a non-rebreather mask by the time you arrive on scene, and has also applied a pulse oximeter that is showing a heart rate of 88 beats/min with SpO_2 levels of 100%. However, when you apply your pulse oximeter to a different finger you are getting a heart rate of 88 beats/min with a SpO_2 reading of 96%.

How can this difference be explained? Which one is correct or incorrect and why would you think so?

ANSWER & DISCUSSION

The accuracy and reliability of pulse-oximetry readings can be affected in various ways, with simple to complex reasons: poor peripheral circulation (due to hypothermia or hypotension), excessive movement, a dirty sensor, interference from ambient ultraviolet light (e.g. sunlight), anaemia or even nail varnish. However, another key factor that can alter these readings is the type of technology the pulse oximeter uses. Most devices within the budget price range utilise a simple infrared light emitter and receiver to measure the levels of haemoglobin with bound molecules (i.e. is there anything attached to the haemoglobin passing through the infrared light?). These cannot differentiate between oxygen and other gases, so they will most likely show 100% when carbon monoxide, such as is present when smoke inhalation occurred, is bound to the haemoglobin. The more advanced pulse oximeters use different wavelengths of infrared light, thus allowing them to differentiate between oxyhaemoglobin and carboxyhaemoglobin, for example, leading to the reading of 96% on your pulse oximeter in this scenario. Hence, the pulse oximeter the CFR is using is most likely indicating a wrong reading and should not be trusted in cases of carbon monoxide inhalation.

CASE 46: ASSESSMENT OF CAPACITY

You are working for the out-of-hours GP service when an ambulance crew calls you to ask for your advice. They are with an elderly patient who is slightly tachypnoeic at 24 breaths/minute and her SpO_2 at 92%. She is pyrexic at 38.7°C and her heart rate is 90 beats/minute. They believe that she has pneumonia, although there are no signs of sepsis, and they would like to convey her to the ED. She is refusing hospitalisation and the crew think that she is a bit confused and would like your advice on assessing her capacity.

What advice would you give on how to assess her capacity?

What would you advise them to do if the patient does not have capacity?

ANSWER & DISCUSSION

The Mental Capacity Act 2005 (MCA) covers the assessment and actions that practitioners should undertake when they are unsure of the patient's capacity to make decisions. Consideration of capacity should not be based on the fact that the patient is deemed to be making an unwise decision. Instead, the assessment of capacity is a two-stage process:

1. Does the patient have an impairment of the mind?
2. Does the impairment mean that the patient is unable to make a specific decision?

This patient would be deemed unable to make this specific decision if she is unable to:

- Understand the information relevant to the decision;
- Retain that information;
- Weigh up that information as part of the decision-making process.

It is important, therefore, to advise that the crew use the points above to assess the patient's capacity. Does she understand the benefits of going to hospital and the risk associated with declining hospital treatment? Is she able to rationalise the decision to you in light of the information that they have given her? If not, she lacks capacity to make this decision. In that case the MCA advises that the practitioner acts in the best interests of the patient, acting in the least restrictive way possible and considering all the relevant circumstances. This might involve discussing with family members or carers in order to consider what might be in the patient's best interests. It seems that in this situation the crew would deem that conveying the patient to hospital would be in her best interests if she lacks capacity to make that decision. The police may be required in order to assist in enacting this management pathway, because the law does allow proportionate restraint to be used. If the patient has capacity to make this decision then it should be respected, no matter how unwise the crew feel it to be. An alternative management plan should be discussed with the patient that is mutually agreeable.

Further resources/recommended reading

MIND, Mental Capacity Act, available at: https://www.mind.org.uk/information-support/legal-rights/mental-capacity-act-2005.

CASE 47: 'NINJAS ON THE LAWN!'

You are called to a private house in an outlying area for a 25-year-old male who reported seeing 'Ninjas on the lawn' in front of his house. The police are also en route and have requested the ambulance service to respond.

What are you thinking when reading this dispatch information? Could this be a valid statement?

The rather comical sound of this dispatch information could easily be mistaken for a practical joke, but that does not make this the most likely answer. As it turns out, the police provide you an update confirming that the patient appears convinced of the presence of ninjas in front of his house, but no unauthorised parties were found by police. You conduct a full primary survey and obtain a full set of vital signs, highlighting no abnormalities, other than a mildly elevated heart rate of 97 beats/minute and a respiratory rate of 24 breaths/minute. Which other vital signs are of particular importance? What are the potential causes of this situation and how can they be uncovered?

ANSWER & DISCUSSION

This patient appears to suffer from delusions or hallucinations, which may have been caused by hallucinogens or other agents that affect the central nervous system. Maintaining an idiosyncratic belief or impression despite events being contradicted by reality or rational argument best defines this type of behaviour, but what are the potential causes?

A thorough history of events reveals that he hosted a party at his house with some friends from his office and that they consumed some 'special brownies' and some 'shrooms', i.e. cannabis brownies and magic mushrooms or a derivative thereof. The evidence of alcohol consumption is also obvious, due to various types of empty bottles and cans spread around the house.

Other vital signs to consider in this context are: 12-lead ECG (to assess for underlying cardiovascular conditions or rhythm disturbances from drug ingestion), as well as pupil size and response (to assess for signs of opioids, stimulants or head injury).

CASE 48: ELDERLY FALLER

An elderly female, aged 78, has fallen in her home and hit her head on a radiator. On your arrival the patient is sitting on her sofa, having managed to get herself off the floor. You undertake a primary survey and find nothing concerning, but you notice obvious swelling and bruising on the right-hand side of the patient's forehead. You ascertain that she fell because she tripped over the edge of a rug, and that there were no concerning symptoms before falling. The patient remembers all of the events: there was no loss of consciousness and, apart from her head being sore, she reports no symptoms. You have no concerns about her cervical spine and inspection of the head confirms that there are no concerns about fractures, either. All of her vital signs are within normal limits.

What would be your management of this patient?

What factors do you need to take into account when forming your management plan?

Is there any other information you need to know to make a decision?

ANSWER & DISCUSSION

This elderly patient has sustained a seemingly minor head injury. In any patient who has sustained a head injury there is a possibility of complications such as intracranial bleeding. To definitively rule out an intracranial bleed a CT scan would be required in hospital. However, it is not practical in terms of resources or in the best interest of the patient to scan every person who has sustained a head injury. Therefore, the paramedic needs to carefully weigh up the risks of complications in this patient. The NICE head injury guidelines give guidance on the types of cases that should be referred to the ED for further assessment or observation. Some key aspects to consider from the history are whether this patient has a history of cerebral haemorrhage or focal neurological symptoms, and whether she is taking anticoagulants. These factors increase the need for her to be monitored in hospital.

It is probably appropriate to discharge this patient on scene, if there is someone who could monitor her for a couple of hours, and on the proviso that they call 999 if she starts to develop abnormal symptoms, such as neurological symptoms.

Further resources/recommended reading

National Institute for Health and Care Excellence (2017) *Head Injury*, London: NICE.

CASE 49: PAEDIATRIC CARDIAC ARREST CALCULATIONS

On the scene of a paediatric cardiac arrest you notice that you forgot your JRCALC pocket book at home and there is no alternative tool in your paediatric bag, such as a Broselow Tape®. During paediatric cardiac arrest management, healthcare professionals rely on weight- and/or height-based pocket books or other tools as a quick and reliable source of drug dosages, airway adjunct sizes and typical vital sign ranges. If these are not available, then the most vital items needed to manage a cardiac arrest have to be calculated. One mnemonic that can be used is W E T Fl A G or W E T F A G, which is made up of the following elements:

W—weight: (age + 4) × 2 = weight in kg

E—energy: 4 joules (J)/kg

T—tube: (age/4) + 4 = inside diameter of endotracheal tube (ET) tube (uncuffed)

Fl or F—fluid (bolus): 20 ml/kg (medical) or 10 ml/kg (trauma)

A—adrenaline: 0.1 ml/kg of 1 mg/10 ml pre-filled syringe adrenaline solution

G—glucose 10% (intravenous solution): 2 ml/kg

This collection of formulae can be used for patients in the age range 1–10 years and, although it is not evidence based, it does provide a reliable way of calculating essential figures needed for cardiac arrest management (Resuscitation Council UK, 2016).

Here are some age groups to practise using the formula:

Patient 1: A 3-year-old boy

Patient 2: A 5-year-old girl

Patient 3: A 10-year-old girl

Once you have completed the calculations, turn to the next page to see the answers.

ANSWER & DISCUSSION

The answers to the drug calculation scenarios on the previous page are as follows:

Patient 1: A 3-year-old boy

Weight: (3 + 4) × 2 = 14 kg

Energy: 4 J × 14 kg = 64 J

Tube: (3 years/4) + 4 = 0.75 + 4 = 4.75 mm internal diameter (ID) (round to the nearest uncuffed tube size)

Fluid: 20 ml × 14 kg = 280 ml (medical) or 10 ml × 14 kg = 140 ml (trauma)

Adrenaline: 0.1 ml × 14 kg = 1.4 ml of 1 mg/10 ml pre-filled syringe adrenaline solution

Glucose: 2 ml × 14 kg = 28 ml of 10% intravenous glucose

Patient 2: A 5-year-old girl

Weight: (5 + 4) × 2 = 18 kg

Energy: 4 J × 18 kg = 72 J

Tube: (5 years/4) + 4 = 1.25 + 4) = 5.25 mm ID (round to the nearest uncuffed tube size)

Fluid: 20 ml × 18 kg = 360 ml (medical) or 10 ml × 18 kg = 180 ml (trauma)

Adrenaline: 0.1 ml × 18 kg = 1.8 ml of 1 mg/10 ml pre-filled syringe adrenaline solution

Glucose: 2 ml × 18 kg = 36 ml of 10% intravenous glucose

Patient 3: A 10-year-old girl

Weight: (10 + 4) × 2 = 28 kg

Energy: 4 J × 28 kg = 112 J

Tube: (10 years/4) + 4) = 2.5 + 4 = 6.5 mm ID (uncuffed tube size)

Fluid: 20 ml × 28 kg = 560 ml (medical) or 10 ml × 28 kg = 280 ml (trauma)

Adrenaline: 0.1 ml × 28 kg = 2.8 ml of 1 mg/10 ml pre-filled syringe adrenaline solution

Glucose: 2 ml × 28 kg = 56 ml of 10% intravenous glucose

Further resources/recommended reading

Resuscitation Council (UK): www.resus.org.uk

CASE 50: FACIAL WEAKNESS

You are working on an ambulance and are passed a call to a 55-year-old male having a possible stroke. You arrive to find the patient sitting on his sofa; he is alert and well perfused. A primary survey reveals no deficits but you do notice that there is obvious facial droop, so you undertake a FAST exam, which reveals the following:

Face—right side of face not moving

Arms—no deficit

Speech—no deficit

Time—you note the time you conducted this exam on your patient care record

The patient reports that he has had some ear pain over the last 24 hours and that his wife noticed his face looked different an hour ago. The patient also feels that he is unable to fully close his right eye and it feels very dry.

What is your preferred diagnosis?

What would be your management of this patient?

ANSWER & DISCUSSION

This patient is suffering from Bell's palsy, which is a unilateral facial nerve paralysis. The exact cause of Bell's palsy is unknown but it appears to be linked to the herpes zoster virus. The facial nerve (cranial nerve XII) becomes paralysed, which affects the lower and upper portion of the face, as opposed to symptoms of a stroke which affect only the lower portion of the face. Therefore, the involvement of the eyelid (patient unable to close his eye) is indicative of a facial nerve paralysis rather than a stroke. In addition, you could ask the patient to raise his eyebrows to show his forehead creases. In Bell's palsy the crease would be lower on the affected side, whereas in a stroke the forehead would not be affected. The fact that this paralysis was preceded by ear pain also adds weight to this diagnosis.

This patient has presented within 72 hours of symptoms starting and therefore should be started on a course of prednisolone. In addition, the patient is unable to fully close his eye so requires lubricating eyedrops to protect the eye. It would be pertinent to refer him to his GP to start this treatment. The patient should be reassured that in most people symptoms resolve within 9 months.

Further resources/recommended reading

National Institute for Health and Care Excellence (2012) *Bell's Palsy*, London: NICE.

CASE 51: COLLAPSE AT THE HARBOUR

The fire service co-responders and your ambulance are sent to the fruit and vegetable cold storage facility at the local harbour for a collapse case. A 39-year-old male staff member is lying on the floor next to an area where fresh fruit is packaged for distribution, on arrival by ship from overseas plantations. He is not alert, is displaying signs of bradypnoea and is pale with signs of emesis around him. After a primary survey he is ventilated with a bag–valve–mask and you notice significant salivation, lacrimation and miosis, as well.

What could be the cause of these signs and symptoms? Which pharmacological intervention is indicated here? How is the location and context of fruit and vegetable import cold storage relevant?

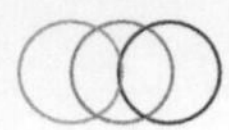

ANSWER & DISCUSSION

Defecation, urination, miosis, bronchospasm, bradycardia, emesis, lacrimation, lethargy and salivation are all typical signs of exposure to organophosphate pesticides and, although these products are banned in the UK and many other countries today, they may still enter the country from countries where they are in use. This is why the cold storage facility for fruit and vegetables is a relevant piece of the history. The patient was exposed to organophosphate residue on the fruit he had been repacking and unloading and, although protective equipment is recommended, there are always instances when this rule may not be meticulously followed, such as in this case.

The key intervention to treat organophosphate exposure is with an anticholinergic agent, such as atropine, in sufficient quantity to achieve a state of atropinisation. This occurs when the cholinergic effects have been sufficiently inhibited, thus reversing all effects of organophosphate poisoning. Due to the strong cholinergic effects, large amounts of atropine are required and the relatively small amounts that are being carried on board ambulances are generally insufficient; 2 mg repeated every 5–10 minutes may have to be repeated dozens of times to achieve the desired result.

Care needs to be taken to prevent exposure of rescuers, but, as the substance is generally not airborne, examination gloves are usually sufficient.

CASE 52: A CHILD WHO FELL

The mother of a 4-year-old girl called 999 saying that her daughter had hurt herself while running around the house today and she thinks she needs to be assessed by a healthcare professional. After a short drive you arrive and find the child sitting on her mother's lap, with clear signs of recent crying, but no visible blood or obvious injuries on approaching her. Utilising the paediatric assessment triangle (PAT) you find the child to be somewhat withdrawn and uninterested in your arrival, but intently focused on her mother, showing no signs of respiratory distress, and she appears to be of a good skin colour.

Jenny, as the mother informs you, was playing inside the house and fell, followed by prolonged crying. She got concerned, because it appeared much louder and unsettling to her, than it normally does. You obtain consent to assess the child and conduct a full primary and secondary survey. While removing her shirt to auscultate the anterior and posterior aspect of the chest, you notice some bruises on the insides of both upper arms, all at different stages of healing, but of similar shape and size. The medical history is unremarkable, except for the course of events, which do not appear to make much sense to you. The mother explains that Jenny had fallen again and that this has happened multiple times before, but this is only the second time an ambulance was called. On trying to find out if she was taken to hospital by ambulance last time, the mother explains that it was decided that transportation to the ED was not necessary last time and she remained at home.

There are no other points of concern, other than the bruising and the history of previous ambulance attendance. Medically you can find no reason to convey Jenny to hospital and the mother is perfectly happy with that decision, but what are some concerns that may have to be addressed here, even if no treatment is undertaken?

ANSWER & DISCUSSION

Not all children with bruises at different stages of healing are required to have a safeguarding referral undertaken, but there is the possibility of a non-accidental injury (NAI) scenario present here. Bruises that are symmetrical, at different stages of healing and do not match the history of events are all possible red flags. Combining this with the refusal of transportation to hospital at the previous incident when an ambulance was called could be a further clue towards this suspicion. A referral is done via either the electronic patient care record system or alternative methods within your place of employment. In cases of immediate danger to the patient, the police may be called upon to remove the child from the environment immediately, but there are no such indications in this case. The key point to keep in mind is that your threshold for reporting should be low, because multiple minor concerns will eventually lead to the identification of trends and, if this turns out not to be a safeguarding concern at all, then that is also not a problem. It is always better to highlight concerns and for them to turn out to be nothing to worry about, than the other way around.

CASE 53: A MAN WITH A SWOLLEN FACE

You are dispatched to a Japanese restaurant for a man with a swollen face who is reportedly struggling to breathe. After a short drive you arrive to find a man in his 30s, sitting in the tripod position in obvious respiratory distress. A waiter from the restaurant is beside the patient with a first-aid kit and an automated external defibrillator (AED) and is looking extremely worried. After a brief introduction you conduct a primary survey and find out the following information:

The patient is alert and fully orientated, but with a distinctly swollen face and tongue. He has a respiratory rate of 26 breaths/minute and an audible inspiratory wheeze. Radial pulses are barely palpable at 104 beats/minute. While you prepare all items needed to immediately address this case of suspected anaphylaxis, your colleague obtains some vital signs:

BP 82/46 mmHg

SpO_2 not giving a reading

3-lead ECG showing a sinus tachycardia at 106 beats/minute

What treatment does this patient require and what is the most important intervention?

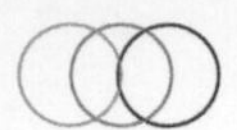

ANSWER & DISCUSSION

Anaphylactic reactions require immediate intervention to prevent detrimental consequences, such as deterioration into cardiac arrest. The first priority is removal of the causative agent and administration of intramuscular adrenaline, 500 mcg into the anterolateral aspect of the thigh. Adrenaline may be repeated every 5 minutes. If not already done, oxygen should now be administered, either via a non-rebreather mask while preparing the nebuliser or immediately via a nebuliser from the start. Salbutamol 5 mg and ipratropium bromide 500 mcg may be combined immediately, but most guidelines recommend attempting monotherapy with only salbutamol first.

Obtaining intravenous access via a large bore cannula (14G or 16G) should follow as soon as possible, because fluid administration is likely to be required. This is due to the increase in vascular permeability through histamine release, which may significantly lower the patient's blood pressure. In this case 0.9% sodium chloride in 250-ml boluses up to 2 litres may be given.

This patient should be transported to the nearest ED as soon as practicable, and they should receive a pre-alert as well. Once the patient can communicate well, i.e. after the adrenaline and other interventions have started to take effect, a history should be taken. Consideration may now also be given to chlorphenamine and hydrocortisone, because they are considered to be beneficial in anaphylaxis cases.

CASE 54: SEVERE BACK PAIN

You are treating a 42-year-old male with severe back pain, while working as a lone responder on a rapid response vehicle. There is no reason or history to suspect a traumatic cause, such as a fall, so spinal immobilisation is not required. He suffered from a 'slipped disc' a few years ago and is now in significant pain after moving some furniture around his apartment. After conducting a primary survey you undertake an OPQRST assessment to gain a better understanding of the pain.

O—pain started while attempting to move a large wardrobe by himself

P—movement makes the pain worse; sitting still relieves it

Q—stabbing pain around the L4 and L5 region of the spine

R—it radiates only a few centimetres around the L4 and L5 area, not anywhere else

S—pain was initially about 7 out of 10, but has now reduced to 5 out of 10 since sitting down

T—all of this started about 40 minutes ago

Managing pain is not an easy undertaking; depending on the circumstances, vital signs, allergies, personal preferences and available drugs the approach may vary significantly.

Which drugs could be used here and how should you decide which analgesic to use?

ANSWER & DISCUSSION

Available options for managing pain within the ambulance service setting can be as simple as positioning the patient or splinting the extremity, and then progress through the stages of oral and inhaled analgesics (paracetamol, codeine, nitrous oxide), escalating to intravenous non-opioid analgesics (intravenous paracetamol), and intravenous and oral opioid analgesics (intravenous and oral morphine). In other words, taking a staggered or stepwise approach to managing pain is the ideal approach.

The main tool in deciding on the appropriate analgesic is the severity of the pain and the preferences of the patient. Morphine should not be used as the first choice for treating mild pain, but it might not be a viable option for severe pain if the patient is refusing intravenous cannulation, either. The World Health Organization designed a pain relief ladder to guide management of pain in cancer patients, but this can also be used as a guide to managing pain in other adult patients, because the focus is on escalating the pain relief from non-opioid in a stepwise fashion to opioid analgesics of different potencies. Currently pain is being managed through positioning and keeping still, but nitrous oxide could be considered as the next step until other options are in place. Intravenous morphine is probably required, especially once transport and manual handling are taking place, but it will possibly not be as effective as it could be. However, the addition of intravenous paracetamol could be the key, because the synergistic effects of morphine and paracetamol have been well documented. This allows the dosage of morphine to be lower, thus reducing the likelihood of potential side effects and improving pain relief.

Further resources/recommended reading

World Health Organization, *Pain Relief Ladder*, available at: www.who.int.

CASE 55: FEVER

You are called to a 4-year-old female whose parents are concerned because she has had a temperature for the last 24 hours, has been coughing a lot and seems generally unwell. You arrive on an RRV and immediately carry out a primary survey. The patient appears to be a good colour, and is not tachypnoeic, not using accessory muscles and alert. You take the following vital signs:

HR 120 beats/minute

RR 27 breaths/minute

SpO_2 98% on room air

Temperature (tympanic) 39.1°C

HGT 5.8 mmol/l

What symptoms/diseases would you want to rule out?

What do you need to take into account when making conveyance decisions?

ANSWER & DISCUSSION

This patient is pyrexic so it is reasonable to assume that she has an infection. Finding the source of the infection would help in determining the severity of the illness. However, there are specific diseases that you would want to rule out, including:

- Meningitis—look for presence of rash, photophobia, neck stiffness neurological symptoms;
- Pneumonia—crackles on auscultation, dyspnoea, low oxygen saturations, accessory muscle use, nasal flaring;
- Urinary tract infection—lethargy, dysuria, urinary frequency, abdominal pain.

It seems that serious illness is absent in this patient, meaning that it is likely that a viral infection is causing these vague symptoms. The presence of a cough may point to a throat or chest infection, which is very likely to be of viral origin. The NICE traffic light system should be used to determine the probable severity of the symptoms and to help guide conveyance decisions. The traffic light system categorises symptoms into green, amber or red depending on their severity. If all symptoms are categorised as green, as is the case for this patient, then she is low risk and it would be suitable to consider discharging on scene. The parents should be advised to keep her well hydrated and to administer paracetamol or ibuprofen to help reduce the symptoms of the infection if required. If there were any amber or red symptoms then referral to the ED should be strongly considered (Figure 2.3). The listed symptoms should help you to identify features for the parents to look out for and to call 999 if any appear.

Further resources/recommended reading

NICE [2013] *Traffic light system for identifying risk of serious illness*. Available from https://www.nice.org.uk/guidance/cg160/resources/support-for-education-and-learning-educational-resource-traffic-light-table-189985789

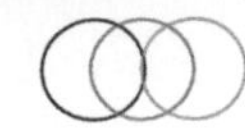

Risk level	Features
High	Ashen, blue or mottled appearance Unresponsive, difficult or impossible to rouse Appears unwell Moderate/severe sternal or intercostal recession Profound tachypnoea Other red flags associated with serious illness (e.g. symptoms of meningitis, sepsis, focal neurological symptoms)
Intermediate	Pale Lethargic Not interacting normally Nasal flaring Oxygen saturations <95% Tachypnoeic Crackles on auscultation
Low	Well perfused Interacting normally Crying normally Perfused and moist mucosa No intermediate or high level risk features of severe illness present

Figure 2.3 Risk levels and features of severe illness

CASE 56: HANGING

A man in his mid-50s is found by passers by in an allotment, after attempting to hang himself in a tree with a rope. He is cut free and bystander cardiopulmonary resuscitation (CPR) is initiated soon after. You arrive at the same time as a community first responder and an ambulance staffed by a paramedic and an ambulance technician. Roles are allocated and advanced life support resuscitation commences. You have been tasked with airway management.

What is your primary concern with regard to airway management? Which options do you have at your disposal/within your scope of practice?

ANSWER & DISCUSSION

Airway management, like most interventions, should be undertaken with the aim to get the most benefit from it, by using the least invasive methods possible. In cases of trauma, particularly around the neck and face, options are not plentiful and timely management of the airway is essential. This patient has potential neck and spinal injuries, so simple manoeuvres like the head-tilt–chin-lift are not an option. Luckily, there are enough staff on scene to assist you with working your way through the stepwise airway management approach (Figure 2.4). Initially, bag–valve–mask ventilation with an oropharyngeal airway might be sufficient, but it is likely that a more invasive approach could become necessary, due to airway oedema, bleeding or haematomas, not to mention the benefit of being able to do asynchronous CPR.

To decrease the chances of a negative outcome from failed airway management strategies, it is beneficial to request a critical care practitioner, HEMS team or other support teams that can undertake a surgical cricothyroidotomy, or even sedate the patient if a return of spontaneous circulation is achieved. Such requests should be done as early as possible and can always be cancelled, if no longer required.

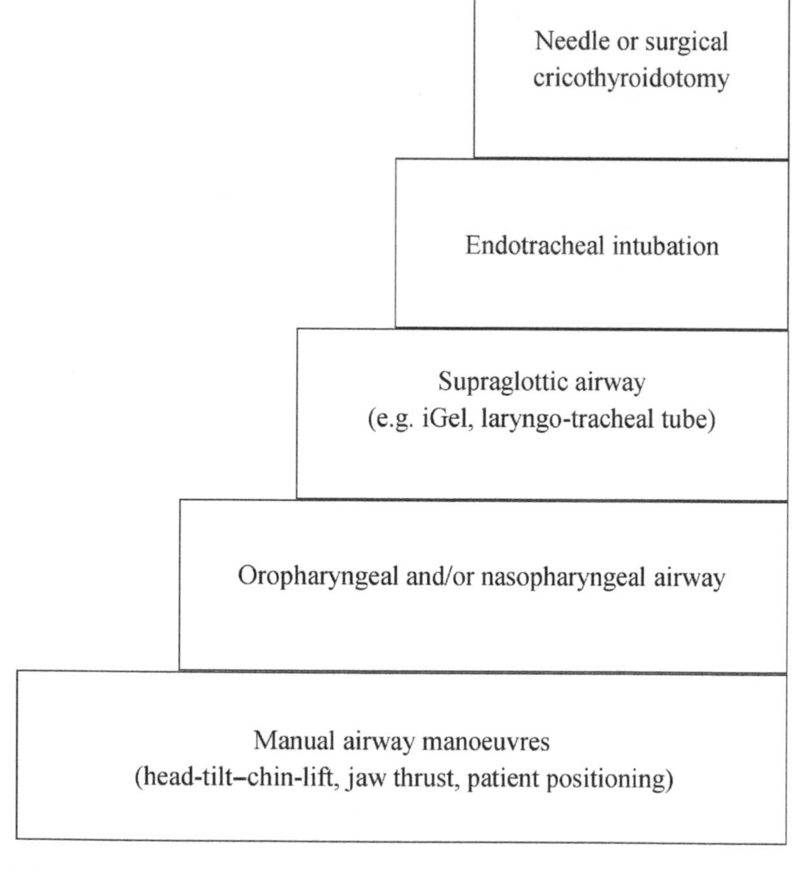

Figure 2.4 Stepwise airway management

CASE 57: KNEE PAIN

Saturday morning, 03:00, you are sent to a 48-year-old female with severe knee pain. A thorough assessment reveals no immediate findings that need to be addressed; the only finding is left-sided, posterior knee pain with some tenderness. Vital signs are all within normal limits and her medical history is as follows:

A—no allergies

M—the pill once a day for the last 10 years; no other medication

P—no medical history other than a caesarean section 20 years ago

L—last urine output at bedtime, last meal was at 20:00 yesterday

E—called 999 after waking up with severe knee pain that did not resolve on its own

Other questions you decide to ask are:

Have you recently travelled by aeroplane or done any scuba diving? No.

Have you been bed bound for long periods recently? No.

Any recent trauma, surgery or previous episodes of knee or leg pain? No.

Why are the answers to these questions relevant? What condition are you trying to rule in or out by asking these questions? What else would you assess the knee for?

ANSWER & DISCUSSION

The reason for asking these questions in addition to the history is to establish if there is the possibility of a DVT (deep vein thrombosis). Air travel, scuba diving, being immobile for extended periods or undergoing surgery can all cause blood clots to form and travel through the systemic circulation, thus leading to a DVT, if within an extremity or a pulmonary embolism (PE), if the clot enters the pulmonary circulation. This patient is not short of breath, has no chest pain and no ECG changes, thus making PE an unlikely diagnosis. Other assessments should include checking for swelling of the knee (posteriorly) and the lower leg, assessing the temperature of the painful area (because it may be much warmer than the rest of the leg) and understanding the relevance of the medication this patient is taking for the last 10 years (i.e. the pill). The contraceptive pill is made up of oestrogen and progesterone, in most cases, and increases the risk for DVT, and being aged over 40 increases the risk even further.

History is the key component in making a diagnosis here, because physical examination can reveal only a certain amount of information and it needs to be combined with physical findings to arrive at a strong differential diagnosis: deep vein thrombosis. This patient should be conveyed to the nearest ED for further examination and treatment, which will most likely include an ultrasound or blood test to confirm the diagnosis, before commencing treatment with anticoagulants.

CASE 58: CONSENT IN MINORS

You are called to a 14-year-old male who has sustained a fractured leg while playing football. When you arrive you assess the patient and identify a fractured mid-shaft tibia and fibula, with no other injuries or concerns. The patient is in a considerable amount of pain and you decide that analgesia is a priority for his patient. You know that your analgesic options are oral paracetamol, oral morphine, intravenous paracetamol and morphine. Your preference is to deliver intravenous morphine so you will need to gain consent to cannulate the patient and to administer it.

The patient is under 16 years of age. Can he consent to these interventions?

What rights do the patient's parents have in overruling the patient's decision?

ANSWER & DISCUSSION

The legal framework that sets out the rights of children aged under 16 years to consent to treatment is called Gillick competence or the Fraser guidelines, and result from a test case in the high court about a minor consenting to contraceptive treatment. The guidelines state that, if the minor has sufficient maturity and intelligence to consent to treatment, can sufficiently weigh up the risks and benefit of a treatment and is free from outside influences such as peer pressure, then a minor may consent to treatment. This is termed 'Gillick competent'. In this case, if the patient can meet the criteria above then he may consent to being cannulated and receiving analgesia. If the patient agrees to consent to treatment and the parents subsequently refuse to consent, then, provided that the patient remains Gillick competent his parents cannot overrule his consent. Gillick competence should be assessed for each decision a minor needs to make. For example, he may be Gillick competent for simple decisions but not have the capacity to understand complex decisions.

If the patient refuses treatment, although he may be assessed as Gillick competent, the parents can consent on the child's behalf. Therefore, Gillick competence is a framework that gives minors the ability to consent to treatment, but parental rights to consent on behalf of the minor are retained if a minor refuses treatment. However, if at all possible it is good practice to discuss all decisions with both the minor and the parents to promote good quality care.

CASE 59: DIVER DOWN

You are called on to respond to the local harbour for a scuba diver who is short of breath, fatigued and complaining of dizziness from about 15 minutes after surfacing from a sea dive with a local diving club. The dive master (DM) has been administering oxygen via a non-rebreather mask since the onset of symptoms about 20 minutes ago, and they commenced the return journey to the harbour, immediately.

Shortly after your arrival at the slipway you establish the following information: the patient is a 39-year-old female with shortness of breath, fatigue, dizziness and generalised muscle weakness, which became blatantly obvious when she tried to climb out of the boat herself and could not support her own weight, despite you and your colleague supporting her on either side. According to the DM she is an experienced diver who undertook only one dive to a depth of 18 m today, lasting about 45 minutes. She is on no regular medication, has no medical history and her vital signs are within normal limits, except for her respiratory rate of 26 breaths/minute (no wheeze or pulmonary oedema present).

Due to the patient being a diver, the environment and the onset you suspect a diving-related condition, such as decompression sickness (DCS) to be the most likely cause. But what are the signs and symptoms of DCS? What treatment is required?

ANSWER & DISCUSSION

DCS may have signs and symptoms appear from as early as during the dive until as much as 12 hours after diving. Colloquially also known as 'the bends', DCS is a consequence of nitrogen being absorbed by the body during the dive, i.e. when at depth, but when surfacing too rapidly the nitrogen does not have sufficient time to be released at a controlled rate so it may form bubbles within tissues and/or the circulatory system, thus causing symptoms. Should these bubbles form in joints, as they often do, then this causes joint pain.

Typical signs and symptoms may include:

- Fatigue of abnormal proportion;
- Itching skin;
- Joint or extremity pain;
- Dizziness;
- Abnormal behaviour, confusion or personality changes;
- Shortness of breath;
- Paralysis or muscle weakness;
- Dysuria;
- Amnesia;
- Cough that may include frothy sputum or blood.

Treatment in a hyperbaric chamber is urgently required for divers suffering from DCS and the control room should be able to contact the nearest hyperbaric chamber or emergency hotline for dive emergencies for you. All patients need to be stabilised before they can be placed in a hyperbaric chamber, so the ED with a pre-alert will be your first stop. Oxygen administration via non-rebreather mask or bag–valve–mask is essential, and intravenous access should be obtained to manage possible dehydration and hypoglycaemia, and maintain end-organ perfusion.

Further resources/recommended reading

Divers Alert Network (DAN): www.diversalertnetwork.org.

CASE 60: ABDOMINAL PAIN

You receive an emergency call to a 75-year-old female with abdominal pain. On arrival she is in obvious pain. She appears slightly pale and sweaty with no issues noted on the primary survey. You take a history from the patient:

HPC: Has had progressively worsening pain since yesterday, got really bad 1 hour ago

S—generalised, slightly worse in left upper quadrant

O—got very severe 1 hour ago

C—sharp in nature

R—radiates all over abdomen, not radiating to back

A—feels very nauseous and is constipated

T—constant

E—nothing makes it better or worse

S—9/10

PMH: Hypertension, previous MI

DHx: Ramipril, clopidogrel, simvastatin

Allergies: None

SHx: Lives with husband; both quite independent

FHx: Nothing significant

ROS: No other issues

All vital signs are within normal limits except the patient is tachycardic at 118 beats/minute.

What are your differential diagnoses?

You undertake an abdominal examination:

Look—there is no obvious distension or discoloration, no scars, no hernias present

Auscultate—there are no bowel sounds present, you cannot hear any bruits

Feel—the left upper quadrant feels hard to touch, there is no pulsating mass

Percuss—the left upper quadrant is dull compared with the left lower quadrant

What is the likely diagnosis and your management plan?

ANSWER & DISCUSSION

The history alone suggests that there may be a significant pathology that should concern you. There are a number of illnesses that could cause such severe pain:

- Appendicitis;
- Pancreatitis;
- Cholecystitis;
- Renal colic;
- Abdominal aortic aneurysm;
- Ruptured bowel;
- Bowel obstruction;
- Constipation.

The history tells us that there is a constant, sharp, generalised pain without pyrexia. With infective causes one would expect pyrexia to be a symptom. Therefore, a number of the above differential diagnoses can be tentatively ruled out. The patient has also had altered bowel movements. The absence of bowel sounds is a red flag for bowel obstruction, and in light of this it would be worth asking if the patient has been able to pass wind; if she has not then there is a complete bowel obstruction. There appears to be a build-up of faeces in the left upper quadrant, suggesting that the bowel obstruction is in the descending colon. This is a surgical emergency requiring analgesia and rapid transport with pre-alert.

CASE 61: SEPSIS

You are treating a patient at a care home who you suspect of having sepsis, caused by a urinary tract infection and repeated episodes of pneumonia and pyrexia. Treatment, aside from conducting a primary and secondary survey for this patient, has to include the Sepsis Six. This treatment regimen includes administration of high-flow (high-concentration) oxygen, taking blood cultures, administering intravenous antibiotics, intravenous fluid resuscitation, checking the lactate level and monitoring hourly urine output; however, not all six interventions are possible within the ambulance service setting, due to the scope of practice of the practitioner, or the unavailability of lactate monitoring or the lack of meeting all indications for treatment within ambulance service practice guidelines.

Assuming that this patient has sepsis, which criteria would he have to meet to be eligible to receive intravenous fluids according to the JRCALC guidelines published in 2017?

ANSWER & DISCUSSION

The JRCALC guidelines are probably the most widely used set of clinical guidelines for paramedics within the UK and generally well known, but present a particular challenge in this case: the indications for intravenous fluid administration in sepsis. JRCALC 2016 required the presence of clinical signs of infection, systolic blood pressure <90 mmHg and tachypnoea; since the update in 2017 tachypnoea is no longer a criterion that needs to be met, allowing paramedics to administer intravenous 0.9% sodium chloride to more sepsis patients than before. Other than the indications, the recommended dosage/volume has not changed. Previously 1 litre every 30 minutes is now 500 ml every 15 minutes, with 2 litres as a maximum dose, just like before. The important aspect to remember is that this fluid resuscitation is for sepsis, not other factors that may have caused dehydration, such as vomiting, diarrhoea or pyrexia, meaning that there is the possibility that more than a total of 2 litres will be required by this patient. Factors such as skin turgor and the moisture level of the mucous membranes need to be taken into consideration, as well.

Further resources/recommended reading

Joint Royal Colleges Ambulance Liaison Committee (2017) *UK Ambulance Services Clinical Practice Guidelines*, London: JRCALC.

National Institute for Health and Care Excellence (2017) *Sepsis*, London: NICE.

CASE 62: MOUNTAIN MEDICINE

You have scheduled your holiday time around a mountaineering expedition to the Himalayas that was looking for volunteers to provide medical support for an independent filmmaking project. Scheduled duration is 2 weeks, a few hours' drive outside of Kathmandu. In preparation you decide to review conditions commonly encountered in mountaineering, particularly at significant altitude and decide to focus on acute mountain sickness (AMS), high altitude pulmonary edema (HAPE) and high altitude cerebral edema (HACE), for today's study and revision session. (The abbreviations are of American origin; as such, the spelling reflects this.)

What do you already know about altitude-related conditions? What are the key pieces of information you think you need to know about? Where would be the best place to find the latest information/guidance?

ANSWER & DISCUSSION

Altitude-related illnesses are not a topic that paramedics tend to be familiar with, particularly in the UK, because the likelihood of occurrence is essentially zero. Therefore, it is essential to familiarise yourself with the altitudes at which these can occur, the signs and symptoms, prevention and treatment options, and where to find the latest treatment advice.

Altitude-related illnesses pose a risk to unacclimatised travellers who ascend to more than 2500m (approximately 8200 feet), but these may occur at altitudes as low as 2000m (approximately 6500 feet). Preventing AMS, HAPE and HACE is best done by limiting ascent rates to 500m of altitude per day (approximately 1600 feet) and may be accompanied by pharmacological prophylaxis with acetazolamide, dexamethasone, nifedipine, tadalafil, sildenafil or salmeterol, depending on the circumstances and risk to the traveller.

Signs and symptoms

Acute mountain sickness (AMS)

- Headache (throbbing, often worsened by lying down).

In addition, at least one of the following:

- Fatigue/exhaustion;
- Loss of appetite, nausea, vomiting;
- Dizziness, feeling light-headed;
- Poor quality of sleep.

High altitude pulmonary edema (HAPE)

- Exhaustion, fatigue, tiredness and a cough;
- Shortness of breath;
- Pulmonary oedema;
- Hypoxia (cyanosis);
- Decreasing level of consciousness as HAPE worsens.

High altitude cerebral edema (HACE)

- Headache (not relieved by NSAIDs or paracetamol);
- Ataxia;
- Decreasing level of consciousness, behavioural changes, hallucinations;
- Nausea and vomiting.

Treatment of altitude illnesses

Treatment must include descent as soon as possible, oxygen administration, avoiding the patient doing exercise by carrying him or her (if at all possible), keeping the patient warm,

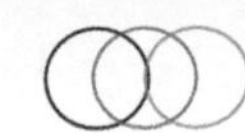

hydrated and maintaining glycaemic control. The patient should be transported and cared for in a position of comfort in order to reduce stress and decrease consequential oxygen demand.

Treatment advice is published by the Wilderness Medical Society (see Further resources/recommended reading, below) and medical screening of candidates before commencement of the expedition is recommended to establish a risk profile for all involved parties, including yourself.

Further resources/recommended reading

Luks, A.M., McIntosh, S.E., Grissom, C.K. et al. (2014) Wilderness Medical Society practice guidelines for the prevention and treatment of acute altitude illness, *Wilderness Environmental Medicine*, 25(4, Suppl), S4–S14.

CASE 63: I'M WORRIED ABOUT MY CREWMATE

You are working with your regular crewmate. You have noticed that over the past couple of weeks he has been more irritable than usual and he seems more distant. You have asked him if everything is OK and he says that he is fine, but you are not so sure. You know that statistically ambulance staff are twice as likely to experience stress at work, but less likely to take time off work, than the general population. You also know that you have been to some traumatic calls recently, including a paediatric cardiac arrest.

What could be wrong with your crewmate?

How might you go about helping him?

ANSWER & DISCUSSION

Your crewmate is displaying signs of stress and/or anxiety. The fact that you have attended traumatic calls recently means that he could be developing post-traumatic stress disorder. Common symptoms of this are:

- Experiencing flashback or intrusive thoughts;
- Emotional numbing;
- Feeling on edge;
- Not sleeping;
- Irritable.

There is support available for mental health issues that arise in the course of a paramedic's work. Your employer should have access to free confidential counselling services and your manager should be able to give you information about this. Alternatively, you can see your GP or self-refer to the NHS talking therapies service in your local area, although waiting times can sometimes be quite long. The charity MIND commenced the 'Blue Light Programme', which gives information to, and offers support services to, emergency service staff who are suffering from a mental health problem. All of the details can be found on their website.

You should try talking to your colleague again. Remember to listen, show empathy and be patient. There may be a culture within the workplace that makes it more difficult to ask for help so acknowledge this but do not put pressure on him. It is also possible that he is experiencing normal stress that we all feel from time to time and that it will pass quickly.

Emergency service workers are at increased risk of developing mental health problems, so it is important that a culture is created where people feel like they can talk about their mental health without stigma.

Further resources/recommended reading

MIND, Blue Light programme, available at: www.mind.org.uk.

CASE 64: PURPLE URINE

An ambulance is requested by a GP to a care home for an 82-year-old female with purple urine bag syndrome (PUBS) for transportation to the nearest hospital. On arrival you are presented with Joanne, a long-term resident of the care home, and her GP who is eagerly awaiting your arrival. Before even taking a handover you notice the unmistakably purple urine in Joanna's urinary drainage bag next to her. According to her GP she has been mostly bed bound for the last year, hence she has had a catheter for almost the entire time, and has also been suffering from constipation and urinary tract infections on a regular basis. The reason for the request for an ambulance today is for further investigation of the purple urine and her abdominal tenderness in the area around the bladder.

After a primary survey you depart the scene towards the nearest hospital and conduct a detailed assessment, finding nothing out of the ordinary other than the points made above.

What is the cause of the purple urine? Which information caused the GP to diagnose PUBS? What treatment will this patient most probably require?

ANSWER & DISCUSSION

Discoloration of urine after catheterisation into a shade of purple is referred to as PUBS (purple urine bag syndrome) and may last from hours to multiple days. The GP diagnosed Joanna based on risk factors for PUBS: chronically catheterised female patients with constipation and potentially elevated urinary bacterial count. All of these apply here and, although the urinary bacterial count has not been evaluated, it is likely to be raised, due to repeated urinary tract infections (UTIs).

PUBS is a rare, but spectacular looking, presentation that occurs when the plastic from a urinary catheter reacts with the metabolites of tryptophan (an amino acid present in many foods and some medication), which is metabolised in the gastrointestinal tract and converted into an indole. This is subsequently converted again, this time by the liver, and mostly excreted into the urine and further digested by some types of bacteria, which turn into blue and red when in contact with alkaline urine, thus creating the distinctive purple colour when it passes through the catheter and into the urine bag, reacting with the above-mentioned plastic. Not all episodes require significant interventions and replacement of the catheter and treatment of the UTI might be all that is required, but this may escalate to sepsis if a UTI is not identified or appropriately treated. There is no particular treatment the ambulance crew can undertake, other than a thorough assessment, including history and vital signs, and being aware of the potential for sepsis.

CASE 65: EXACERBATION OF COPD

You are called to a 76-year-old male with an acute exacerbation of chronic obstructive pulmonary disease (COPD). On arrival he is breathless, using accessory muscles, and appears pale and diaphoretic. You undertake a primary survey and find a global expiratory wheeze with dyspnoea. While your crewmate sets up a salbutamol nebuliser with oxygen you take the following vital signs:

HR 120 beats/minute and regular, radial pulse present

RR 30 breaths/minute

BP 145/75 mmHg

SpO_2 84% on room air

HGT 5.6 mmol/l

Temperature (tympanic) 38.9°C

Once the patient has been nebulised with salbutamol you can see that he looks much less breathless; this is the second set of vital signs:

HR 90 beats/minute and regular, radial pulse present

RR 20 breaths/minute

BP 147/77 mmHg

SpO_2 92% on room air

HGT 5.7 mmol/l

Temperature (tympanic) 38.8°C

On auscultation you can hear very minor expiratory wheeze and crackles in the right lower lobe. He is no longer using accessory muscles and feels like he is breathing much more easily. He tells you that he usually has a cough but it has worsened over the last couple of days, and he has been producing green sputum, which he does not normally.

What is your management of this patient?

ANSWER & DISCUSSION

This patient has an infective exacerbation of COPD. It is likely that he has pneumonia because of the crackles on auscultation, his raised temperature and the sputum that he is producing. He has responded well to a salbutamol nebuliser and, provided that he stays well saturated when not on oxygen, he could be safely discharged at home.

Salbutamol is short acting so, in order to decrease the risk of the symptoms worsening over the next couple of hours, you should arrange for him to commence a 5- to 7-day course of oral steroids. Steroids generally suppress the immune response and may augment the effect of salbutamol, which will hopefully stop the symptoms returning.

It is important to treat the cause of the exacerbation, which in this case is a chest infection, probably pneumonia. The patient should be commenced on a course of antibiotics, the choice of which will be guided by local resistance and whether he has a specific antibiotic that usually works for his chest infections (if he has had this before).

The patient should be referred to his general practitioner to follow up on him, and he should be informed that if the symptoms return he should call 999.

Further resources/recommended reading

National Institute for Health and Care Excellence (2010) *COPD in Over 16s*, London: NICE.

CASE 66: EPIGASTRIC PAIN

A 56-year-old female complaining of abdominal pain originating just below the xiphoid process is being attended by yourself and your colleague. The vital signs and history can be summarised as follows:

Vital signs

HR 82 beats/minute

RR 18 breaths/minute

SpO_2 of 97% on room air

BP 130/72 mmHg

HGT 5.7 mmol/l

Temperature (tympanic) 37.7 C

12-lead ECG: Normal sinus rhythm

History

Allergies: Lamb's wool

Medication: Omeprazole (for gastric reflux)

Past medical history: Gallstones, paracetamol for occasional back pain

Last input/output: Two cans of lager for dinner and two for lunch; last urinated and defecated about an hour ago

Events: Severe pain in the epigastric region made her call 999 tonight

Pain assessment

O—sudden onset about 2 hours ago

P—pain is mildly alleviated by assuming the fetal position; nothing alleviates the pain

Q—stabbing pain

R—radiates to the back

S —8 out of 10

T—continuous pain since about 2 hours ago

Besides the abdominal pain she is also complaining of nausea, but she has not vomited today. The abdominal exam reveals moderate tenderness in the left and right upper quadrants. You are not completely certain after palpating the abdomen that there is some mild distension present, so you include this finding in your notes and decision-making process.

Which condition is the most likely diagnosis here? Which analgesic(s) could you administer to manage her pain?

ANSWER & DISCUSSION

This patient most probably suffers from acute pancreatitis, based on the history of gallstones, suspected regular alcohol consumption and stabbing abdominal pain. Alleviation of the pain when assuming the fetal position and the presence of abdominal distension, even if only minor, are further diagnostic clues. Acute pancreatitis is the inflammation of the pancreas and may be classified as mild (no complications and full recovery), moderate (localised complications and resolves within 48 hours) or severe (organ dysfunction with failure to resolve in 48 hours). At this stage you could classify this case of acute pancreatitis as either moderate or severe, but the final verdict will depend on the remaining timeframe of symptoms. Pain management may include any of the available options within your scope of practice, such as NSAIDs, paracetamol, nitrous oxide or even morphine, assuming there are no contraindications present.

Once the patient reaches the ED lipase or amylase levels will be tested to confirm the diagnosis and imaging studies may also be undertaken. In addition, it is likely that another 12-lead ECG and cardiac marker test will be undertaken to rule out a myocardial infarction as the cause of the pain.

Further resources/recommended reading

National Institute for Health and Care Excellence (2016) *Pancreatitis—Acute*, London: NICE.

CASE 67: DISPLACED PATELLA

You are called to a 21-year-old male who bystanders say has 'broken his kneecap'. You arrive to find the patient who looks alert and a good colour but is in a lot of pain. He is holding his right leg with his knee bent at 90°. You undertake a primary survey and find no deficits. You see that the right patella has been displaced laterally. The patient tells you that he had his weight on his right leg when he turned and felt his knee 'pop'; there was no other impact.

What would be your management of this patient?

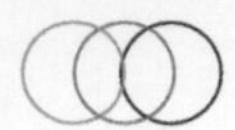

ANSWER & DISCUSSION

The patient has displaced his patella laterally as a result of a turning motion, and the history suggests that there has been no other traumatic impact. You should first make sure that there is no nerve or vascular damage distal to the injury, by checking sensation and colour of the foot, although this is unlikely to have occurred in this injury.

The patient is in a lot of pain and requires analgesia. Nitrous oxide and oxygen (Entonox) is a good choice of analgesia because you are planning to relocate the patient's patella, which will severely reduce the pain in itself, so stronger analgesia is probably not required.

To relocate the patella you will first need to ensure that the Entonox is having the maximum effect possible and then straighten the patient's right leg, while applying pressure on the displaced patella towards the normal anatomical position. Before the leg straightens fully the patella should relocate.

Once relocated, the pain should decrease substantially and the patient may be transported to the ED for review and further referral.

CASE 68: 'THERE IS BLOOD EVERYWHERE!'

The police and your ambulance are sent to an apartment of an elderly woman, after the carer called 999, because 'There is blood everywhere, please come quickly'. As the origin of the blood has not yet been established it is a possibility that this is an active crime scene.

You are met by a police officer at the door to the apartment who explains to you that the scene is safe and that it appears to be a medical emergency, because the patient is bleeding from her right leg. A fellow officer has already controlled the bleeding with a pressure dressing and introduces you to Marjorie, the 84-year-old resident. Her carer who comes in twice a day to look after her is also present. Your colleague takes some vital signs while you get a medical history from the carer: no allergies; takes digoxin for atrial fibrillation (AF); has cataracts and reduced visual acuity, but is mobile with the aid of a walker and lives alone with her dog, Dave.

Vital signs

HR 94 beats/minute and mildly irregular

SpO_2 98% on room air

BP 135/50 mmHg

12-lead ECG shows a sinus rhythm with AF

An examination of the leg reveals obviously visible veins, with the injured section located half-way between the knee and ankle. Coincidentally this matches the height of the blood spatter all around the apartment and on her dog.

What is the diagnosis here? What treatment is required, if any?

ANSWER & DISCUSSION

The diagnosis is varicose veins, which are superficial, dilated veins on the legs that mostly cause no concern to most patients, other than their appearance. To others, minor trauma to the legs, such as from bumping against furniture or while undertaking daily tasks, may result in significant bleeding. In this case, Marjorie, due to her reduced visual acuity, must have injured her leg in her apartment, but was not able to see the bleeding, so she consequentially did nothing about it. It was only her carer who noticed and called 999. Management, other than controlling the bleeding, should be followed up with a referral to a vascular service/specialist. Taking Marjorie to the ED is probably not required, unless systemic signs of shock or other concerns are present, but arrangements should be made with her carer to arrange for a consultation as soon as possible.

Further resources/recommended reading

National Institute for Health and Care Excellence (2014) *Varicose Veins*, London: NICE.

CASE 69: 'DID I MAKE A MISTAKE?'

You just finished a night shift during which you attended to a 26-year-old female with an anaphylactic reaction to shellfish at a restaurant. On your way home you listen to a radio show where allergic reactions are discussed and the role adrenaline administration plays in such cases. Then it occurs to you: Did I administer the whole ampoule of adrenaline in one go or did I administer 500 mcg followed by 500 mcg 5 minutes later? A mild panic starts to set in as you are going through the whole case in your head.

Who do I need to inform about this? Do I need to report this to the Health and Care Professions Council (HCPC) as a self-referral case? Will I lose my registration with the HCPC?

ANSWER & DISCUSSION

The first thing you should do is get in touch with your line manager to express your concern that you may have made a clinical mistake, because this is currently only a suspicion. At this stage it is not yet of concern to the HCPC, because it is your duty to complete a self-referral only if there are restrictions placed on your practice, or if you are suspended or dismissed by your employer for improper conduct or concerns about your clinical competence. Your line manager will probably complete some reporting paperwork and then review case records of the above-mentioned incident. Should your suspicion of a clinical error not be true, than this will be the end of this investigation. If not, then an internal process will be followed that may include a review of all paperwork, speaking to colleagues and you being invited to a review panel. Once this is completed the decision may be that you are required to attend some further training, work under supervision or simply get a written warning issued to you and placed in your file.

Your registration does not have to be affected at all and the HCPC encourages employers and registrants to deal with potential cases of concern within their practice setting first, before escalating this to the HCPC.

Further resources/recommended reading

Health and Care Professions Council (2017) *People like us? Understanding complaints about paramedics and social workers*, London: HCPC.

Health and Care Professions Council (2016) *Standards of Conduct, Performance and Ethics*, London: HCPC.

CASE 70: COLLAPSE

On a hot summers day you respond to a church for a collapse case. You are first on scene at the rather crowded church, with an elderly congregation member lying on the ground, surrounded by numerous people.

After having created some space around the patient you introduce yourself to an alert and orientated female named Catherine, aged 60, who says she is sorry for having called you for this because she is fine now. She was attending the church service and was standing at the back, due to no free seats, when she collapsed just before the end of the service. You explain to her that you would like to assess her, just to be sure she is okay, to which she agrees.

Vital signs

HR 68 beats/minute

RR 18 breaths/minute

SpO_2 of 97% on room air

BP 140/80 mmHg

3-lead ECG showing normal sinus rhythm

HGT 4.9 mmol/l

Temperature (tympanic) 36.1°C

FAST exam negative

The physical exam reveals no physical injuries and no incontinence, and the history highlights no areas of concern, either.

What is the most likely diagnosis? Which other assessments should be undertaken? Does Catherine have to go to hospital?

ANSWER & DISCUSSION

The short duration of the loss of consciousness, absence of incontinence, hypoglycaemia or a history of epilepsy, combined with prolonged standing in a rather warm environment are suggestive of syncope ('blackout'), also referred to as transient loss of consciousness (TLoC). To confirm this diagnosis, a 12-lead ECG to rule out a cardiac cause should also be undertaken.

Specialist referral is indicated in the presence of an abnormal ECG, history or signs of heart failure, exertional TLoC, family cardiac history, or shortness of breath with no identifiable cause or a murmur. Patients aged >65 years should also be referred if no prodromal symptoms, such as sweating or feelings of hot and cold, are the likely context.

Patients with a TLoC should be taken to the ED unless it is confirmed to be situational syncope or uncomplicated faint. Catherine is not, however, meeting the criteria for admission or referral and can be safely discharged on scene. Accurate documentation of all assessments is essential, as always.

Further resources/recommended reading

National Institute for Health and Care Excellence (2014) *Transient Loss of Consciousness ('Blackouts') in Over 16s*, CG109, London: NICE.

CASE 71: VOMITING AND LETHARGY

You are dispatched to a 38-year-old male with persistent vomiting and lethargy. He called 999 himself and, while you introduce yourself and obtain some further information about the preceding events, he vomits. After your assessment the vital signs and history are as follows:

HR 92 beats/minute and regular

RR 18 breaths/minute

SpO_2 of 96% on room air

BP 90/50 mmHg

HGT 21.6 mmol/l

3-lead ECG showing normal sinus rhythm

Allergies: None

Medication: None

Past medical history: Tonsillectomy 6 years ago

Last meal/last output: Two chocolate bars as a snack 2 hours ago; frequent urination

Events: Persistent lethargy for the last 24 hours or more; frequent vomiting started a few hours ago and he feels like he has to urinate a lot

What is your differential diagnosis? Which specific treatment is needed?

ANSWER & DISCUSSION

This patient is suffering from diabetic ketoacidosis (DKA), which is a metabolic disorder that is a consequence of relative or absolute insulin deficiency, resulting in hyperglycaemia, acidaemia and ketosis. Diagnosis is based on three criteria mentioned above: glucose >11.0 mmol/l or a history of diabetes mellitus, presence of ketones ≥3.0 mmol/l 3.0 mmol/l or more than 2+ on standard urine dipsticks and acidosis, with a pH <7.3 and/or serum bicarbonate <15 mmol/l, but all except the serum glucose and urine dipstick values cannot be easily assessed in the ambulance service setting.

Treatment must include oxygen if SpO_2 is <94%, but this is not the case here. Specific treatment for DKA in this patient means intravenous 0.9% sodium chloride to restore circulatory volume, aid the clearance of ketones and correct any electrolyte imbalance. Intravenous insulin will be administered by ED staff on arrival in hospital to suppress ketogenesis and reduce blood glucose levels.

The typical fluid deficit in DKA in adults is around 100 ml/kg for water alone, so the likelihood of causing harm by rehydrating liberally is fairly low. A typical 75-kg patient would therefore require about 7500 ml (7.5 litres) of intravenous fluids. However, care needs to be taken to avoid causing cerebral oedema, although most guidelines, such as those of the JRCALC, limit intravenous fluid administration to 2 litres for the treatment of DKA, so this risk should be very low.

Further resources/recommended reading

British Diabetes Society (2013) *Management of Diabetic Ketoacidosis in Adults*, London: British Diabetes Society.

Joint Royal Colleges Ambulance Liaison Committee (2017) *UK Ambulance Services Clinical Practice Guidelines*, London: JRCALC.

CASE 72: DIARRHOEA

Around 07:30 on a Saturday morning, you and your colleague are dispatched to a 34-year-old female with diarrhoea. The initial assessment reveals no abnormalities, i.e. she is alert and orientated, has equal, bilateral, clear air entry and strong radial pulses. You take some vital signs while your colleague obtains a history. The patient started taking amoxicillin yesterday evening (Friday) after being diagnosed with an ear infection by her GP at around 18:00. She developed diarrhoea during the course of the night and started feeling 'like she has a fever'. Reviewing the medication packet you establish that she was prescribed 500 mg every 8 hours for otitis media for 5 days. She has no allergies and is taking no medication, other than occasional sinus relief tablets for sinusitis (over-the-counter medication).

All her vital signs are within normal limits, but her tympanic temperature is slightly elevated at 37.8°C.

What is the most likely cause of this case of diarrhoea? What could the patient do to prevent dehydration and electrolyte imbalances from diarrhoea?

ANSWER & DISCUSSION

Antibiotics-related side effects are very common in penicillin-based antibiotics, and may include diarrhoea, fever, rashes and urticaria. Therefore, diarrhoea and fever in an otherwise stable and healthy patient are most probably caused by the amoxicillin and are not a significant concern. As the patient assessment revealed no signs of an allergic reaction, discharge of this patient at home is the safe and recommended choice. Oral rehydration therapy (ORT) is designed to replace electrolytes and fluids lost from diarrhoea and are available as numerous over-the-counter products, but maintaining a normal diet and adequate fluid intake will often provide the same benefits.

Acute diarrhoea tends to be self-limiting in 2–4 days, but in the case of penicillin-induced diarrhoea it is possible that it could last as long as the course of antibiotics (5 days in this case). A consultation with the GP should be undertaken if it has not improved by Monday morning, although it is likely to have improved by then.

CASE 73: FEMALE UNRESPONSIVE

A female in her mid-20s is found unresponsive by her flatmates and they call 999 immediately. After a 7-minute ambulance response you arrive on scene. According to her flat mates, Claire was feeling very tired the whole afternoon and decided to get some fresh air by going for a run. Claire laid down for a nap afterwards, but her flatmates could not wake her. When you arrive you immediately start a primary survey and establish the following:

- Only responsive to pain on the AVPU scale;
- Airway open and maintained by herself (oropharyngeal airway [OPA] not tolerated);
- RR 14 breaths/minute;
- HR 60 beats/minute and regular (radial pulses present);
- SpO_2 of 92% on room air, so you immediately apply oxygen via a non-rebreather mask;
- 3-lead ECG showing a normal sinus rhythm;
- HGT 1.7 mmol/l;
- Skin is pale, cold and clammy.

Claire is clearly hypoglycaemic and her flat mates mention to you that she has been eating very little lately, because she is trying to lose some weight to allow her to fit into her dream wedding dress by next week.

What are your treatment options for hypoglycaemia? Which pharmacological intervention should be avoided?

ANSWER & DISCUSSION

Hypoglycaemia can occur in any person, not only diabetics. In Claire's case, dieting by reducing her overall calorie input combined with physical activity is the most probable cause for her hypoglycaemic episode. Seeing that she was already feeling tired before her run indicates that her blood glucose level was probably already low before she did her exercise. Due to this, glucagon is not likely to be a good choice for managing hypoglycaemia, even if intravenous access fails, because her glycogen stores are likely to be depleted. Intravenous 10% glucose is the best and most rapidly acting pharmacological intervention and should be your first choice. Alternatively, oral glucose gel may be applied to a gauze swab and placed between Claire's cheek and teeth to allow for absorption without significant risk of aspiration. Ideally she should be in the lateral position while glucose gel is being administered this way.

CASE 74: PATIENT FEELING UNWELL

John, a 59-year-old male who is feeling unwell, is the first patient you attend to on your shift today. He is a known cardiac patient and has been on various medications over recent years, and it is not the first time you have been called to him. During your assessment you discover bradycardia and hypotension.

Looking at his current and previous list of medications you come across the following generic names:

- Metoprolol;
- Diltiazem;
- Amlodipine;
- Atenolol;
- Verapamil.

Assuming the bradycardia and hypotension are caused by one of his medications at an inappropriately high dosage, what type/class of medications are the ones mentioned above? Which diagnostic test(s) would enable you to identify the causative drug type/class? What treatment is likely to be required or should be considered?

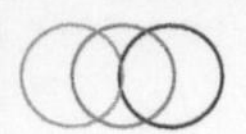

ANSWER & DISCUSSION

The two types/classes of drugs that John has been on are beta blockers (metoprolol and atenolol) and calcium channel blockers (diltiazem, amlodipine, verapamil). Due to their common pharmacological properties, despite different mechanisms, hypotension and bradycardia are common side effects. One diagnostic test that allows you to differentiate between these two classes of drugs is a haemo-gluco-test. Patients with a calcium channel blocker overdose are generally hyperglycaemic, whereas beta-blocker overdoses have no effect on blood glucose levels.

Treatment, other than oxygen via a non-rebreather mask and airway management, may include: intravenous fluid therapy (0.9% sodium chloride), atropine to manage bradycardia not resolved by oxygenation and intravenous fluid administration, and may also include insulin. Potentially, activated charcoal may also be an option, if it can be safely administered to the patient (i.e. no decreased level of consciousness and less than one hour has elapsed since ingestion).

Beta-blocker overdoses are treated in the same way, but may include glucagon as an additional pharmacological intervention. Its efficacy is, however, not well documented and may cause adverse effects.

Further resources/recommended reading

British National Formulary, Emergency treatment of poisoning, (in print, via the smartphone app or via www.medicinescomplete.com).

National Poisons Information Service: www.npis.org.

TOXBASE: www.toxbase.org.

CASE 75: 'MY MOTHER SUFFERS FROM DEPRESSION'

You and your colleague are sent to a 68-year-old female who is reportedly behaving abnormally. On arrival her daughter meets you at the door and directs you to the living room. She explains that Maria, her mother, is suffering from depression and that she is taking 60 mg of clomipramine hydrochloride once a day, but has been very restless and agitated today.

After a conversation and detailed assessment you agree with the initial impression of Maria's behaviour and have found out the following information:

- Maria is alert, but visibly restless, euphoric and agitated;
- Her skin appears flushed;
- She has a dry mouth and a headache;
- HR 126 beats/minute;
- RR 20 breaths/minute;
- SpO_2 of 96% on room air;
- Temperature (tympanic) 37.8 C;
- 12-lead ECG showing sinus tachycardia with wide QRS complexes at a rate of 126 beats/minute.

History

Allergies: None

Medication: Clomipramine hydrochloride 60 mg once daily

Past medical history: Depression since 2010 after her husband died

Last meal/output: Lunch about an hour ago; she has not urinated in about 8 hours

Events: Feeling agitated and restless since this morning

Looking at the vital signs and history, what is the likely diagnosis? What treatment specific to this condition is needed?

ANSWER & DISCUSSION

Maria is suffering from a tricyclic antidepressant (TCA) overdose. Signs and symptoms include dry mouth, tachycardia, urinary retention, restlessness, euphoria, hyperthermia and ECG changes (QRS widening beyond 120 ms in this case). TCAs have a narrow therapeutic window, so over- or under-dosing are easily possible, which is how Maria ended up with an overdose. There is no antidote for a TCA overdose, but certain elements beyond maintaining airway, breathing and circulation should be included. This should include continuous ECG monitoring to allow for early detection of dysrhythmias and recognition of cardiac arrest, administration of activated charcoal if less than an hour has elapsed since ingestion, sodium bicarbonate to aid with reduction of toxicity and cardiac dysrhythmias (if within your scope of practice), and potentially diazepam for treating seizures.

Maria requires a toxicological assessment in the ED and should be monitored for multiple hours after becoming asymptomatic. However, before this stage is reached she might require benzodiazepines to manage her agitation, should this become a concern.

Further resources/recommended reading

British National Formulary, Emergency treatment of poisoning, (in print, via the smartphone app or via www.medicinescomplete.com)

National Poisons Information Service: www.npis.org.

TOXBASE: www.toxbase.org.

CASE 76: VOMITING BLOOD

At 05:00 a 58-year-old male calls 999 for an ambulance after he starts to vomit blood. After only a 5-minute response time you and your colleague arrive on scene. Roger meets you at the door, holding a bucket. He has lightly bloodshot eyes and appears quite pale, but is fully alert and orientated. His vital signs are all within normal limits for an adult of his age.

Roger has no allergies and takes aspirin (acetylsalicylic acid) 75 mg once daily, as well as omeprazole once a day. He had a myocardial infarction in 2008, but no other medical history. Passing urine and stool have been normal and his last meal was a microwaveable meal from the local petrol station he at about 02:00. When asked about the events of last night he explains that he went to a friend's stag do, had quite a lot to drink and then took a taxi home. After eating the microwave meal he went to bed, but at about 04:30 he woke up and vomited violently. Since then he has vomited multiple times and seen blood mixed into it and been feeling nauseated.

What is your diagnosis and would you have to take Roger to hospital?

ANSWER & DISCUSSION

Roger is hung over after drinking excessively, but also suffering from Mallory–Weiss syndrome, a condition affecting the oesophagus at the level of the stomach, causing tears that can be 1- to 4-cm long which lead to arterial bleeding. Severity can range from mild to life threatening, and may trigger further vomiting if sufficient amounts of blood are swallowed. Roger has not vomited since you arrived, but his earlier violent episodes of vomiting were sufficiently powerful to create an oesophageal tear, leading to blood in his vomit. Risk factors include prolonged aspirin use and excessive alcohol intake, both of which he meets. He is not a known alcoholic, but the excessive drinking of the night before increased his risk significantly. Hospitalisation is not required, unless his vital signs and frequency of vomiting were to worsen. He should be advised to call 999 again, if he does not feel better in a few hours, or if the amount of blood in his vomit increases.

CASE 77: ABDOMINAL PAIN

On a Friday evening you are dispatched to an Indian restaurant for a patient with severe abdominal pain. You are shown to a side room of the restaurant where a female in her late 40s is sitting by a table, holding her abdomen and appearing to be in significant pain. Before you manage to introduce yourself and get any assessments done the patient vomits. Now you manage to speak with her and find out what happened. Becky, the patient, was having an end-of-year function with her colleagues at this restaurant, when about 30 minutes after the meal she started to get severe abdominal pain.

Her vital signs included a heart rate of 98 beats/minute, respiratory rate of 20 breaths/minute, SpO_2 of 97% on room air and a pain score of 8 out of 10. During the physical examination you identify the location of the pain as the right upper quadrant, superiorly. There is no rebound tenderness present, reducing the likelihood of appendicitis, and the history reveals nothing of concern, such as recent surgery, alcoholism or a missed menstrual period, which could lead to the differential diagnosis of ectopic pregnancy.

What is the diagnosis and what treatment is required?

ANSWER & DISCUSSION

Cholecystitis is inflammation of the gallbladder which may result in obstruction of the bile duct. Consequentially, particularly after a greasy meal, a lot of bile is required to break down the fat, so, as the food passes from the stomach to the duodenum, the gallbladder releases bile and due to the inflammation causes significant pain. Chest pain of cardiac origin needs to be considered as a potential differential diagnosis, so a 12-lead ECG and OPQRST assessment of the pain are required. Other differential diagnoses may include gastric reflux and oesophageal spasm.

Treatment is initially merely symptomatic until the diagnosis can be confirmed with imaging studies and the gallbladder can be surgically removed. This includes maintaining the fluid balance with intravenous 0.9% sodium chloride, providing analgesia and administration of an antiemetic, if required.

Further resources/recommended reading

National Institute for Health and Care Excellence (2017) *Cholecystitis—Acute*, London: NICE.

CASE 78: HYPERPIGMENTATION

A 38-year-old female presents to the GP surgery you are working at today, complaining of fatigue, weight loss, joint and abdominal pain, and hyperpigmentation.

Before taking her vital signs you speak to her about the progress of her fatigue and other symptoms. She explains that she has been feeling lethargic and exhausted basically every day for at least 2 months now, and that she has been losing weight without changing her diet. Recently, she also noticed that she had regular abdominal pain, not just during her menstrual cycles, and that her hands and some skin creases on her body appear to be getting darker.

Her blood pressure is 100/60 mmHg while sitting, but 80/50 mmHg after standing up and associated with some mild dizziness.

What is the most likely diagnosis and how should this be treated?

ANSWER & DISCUSSION

Addison's disease is the suspected diagnosis here, because it is characterised by fatigue, hyperpigmentation, weight loss, joint and abdominal pain, and postural dizziness caused by hypotension. These signs and symptoms are caused by adrenal cortex insufficiency, which are responsible for the production of multiple hormones, including adrenaline, aldosterone and cortisol, and are located on both kidneys.

Treatment in this scenario is not an emergency, because the patient is not displaying signs of hypotension, hypovolemic shock, acute abdominal pain, low-grade fever or vomiting, but should be investigated and treated regardless. Referral to an endocrinologist should be considered, but cortisol levels should be established by sending blood samples off to the lab to confirm the diagnosis. Glucocorticoid therapy is the most commonly used option and drugs such as hydrocortisone can be taken orally by the patient, often in three daily doses to mimic the natural release cycle. To prevent deterioration into an Addisonian crisis, 100 mg of intramuscular hydrocortisone may be administered by paramedics, even if there is doubt about the diagnosis.

Further resources/recommended reading

National Institute for Health and Care Excellence (2016) *Addison's Disease*, London: NICE.

CASE 79: ASSESSING A PATIENT'S GLASGOW COMA SCALE SCORE

Assessment of the neurological status of patients has numerous elements, but one that often leads to varying degrees of results is the Glasgow Coma Scale (GCS), because the interpretation or level of competence with the GCS varies. Eye opening is scored out of 4 points, verbal response out of 5 points, motor response out of 6 points, with a maximum score of 15 out of 15.

The following scenarios give you the opportunity to test your knowledge without having the GCS in front of you. How many points does each patient score on the GCS?

Patient A: Eyes open spontaneously; he is confused and localises pain.

Patient B: Eyes open on painful stimulus; she makes incomprehensible sounds and withdraws from pain.

Patient C: Eyes open to speech; responses to questions vary between confused and orientated in the same sentence and he withdraws from pain.

Turn to the next page to see the answers.

ANSWER & DISCUSSION

Here are the answers for the patients above:

Patient A: Eyes 4; verbal 4; motor 5 = 14 out of 15

Patient B: Eyes 2; verbal 2; motor 4 = 8 out of 15

Patient C: Eyes 3; verbal 4 or verbal 5; motor 4 = 11 or 12 out of 15

Patient C is the only one where the question arises of which answer is the most correct one, because he varies between confused and orientated in the same sentence. So which score should you use as your baseline and document on your patient care record?

Use 12 out of 15, because the GCS is based on the patient's best response in each category, not the worst.

Further resources/recommended reading

Teasdale, Sir G.M. (2014) The Glasgow Structured Approach to Assessment of the Glasgow Coma Scale, available at: www.glasgowcomascale.org.

CASE 80: BLOOD SUGAR DERAILMENT

On a long bank-holiday weekend you are dispatched to a 68-year-old female who called 999, because her blood sugar is 'abnormal'. You arrive on your own on the rapid response vehicle and locate the address without any delays. Elizabeth, the patient, meets you at the door, thanks you for coming so quickly and explains to you on the way to the living room that she tested her blood sugar and it 'just isn't right'.

Following a brief primary survey to assess for any immediately life-threatening presentations you obtain a full set of vital signs:

HR 72 beats/minute and regular

RR 14 breaths/minute

SpO_2 of 98% on room air

BP 145/80 mmHg

Temperature (tympanic) 36.7 C

3-lead ECG showing a normal sinus rhythm

HGT 4.2 mmol/l

Her medical history is as follows:

Allergies: Asparagus

Medication: Multi-vitamins, paracetamol for occasional headaches, metformin once a day

Past medical history: Non-insulin-dependent diabetes mellitus

Last meal/output: Tea and biscuits at breakfast time; urine output about an hour ago

Events: She called 999, because her blood sugar was abnormal; when asked what she means by that, she has no sensible answer

Judging by her vital signs and history, there appears to be nothing significantly abnormal happening here. What could be going on? What types of questions would you like to ask her to help you identify the real reason for calling 999 today?

ANSWER & DISCUSSION

Elizabeth does not appear to have 'abnormal' blood sugar readings, as she claimed on the phone to 999, nor does she have any abnormal vital signs or elements of her history, other than her inability to explain her concerns about the blood sugar readings. The environment should be considered in this scenario. Does it look like she cannot look after herself? Are there clues that could point you towards an alternative cause for calling 999?

Looking around you identify what appears to be a patient care record from the ambulance service. Elizabeth gives you permission to read it and then admits that she did not actually test her blood sugar before she called. The patient care record tells a similar story to today, no abnormalities found during the examination and history, and no conveyance to hospital. On the way to the lounge, you also noticed a lot of family pictures on the walls, but none that appears particularly recent. You then take the opportunity to explore her social history and it turns out that she has been living alone since her husband died 6 years ago, and that she has four grandchildren whom she has not seen in over a year.

Loneliness is obviously the motivating factor for Elizabeth to call the ambulance service twice in recent times, so preventing future calls by providing some advice to her is a good idea.

Potential avenues to explore are:

> The Silver Line, a helpline for older people: 0800 4 70 80 90 (www.thesilverline.org.uk)
>
> Age UK, a charity that supports elderly people with free advice on healthcare, money, loneliness and wellbeing: 0800 169 8787 (www.ageuk.org.uk)

CASE 81: PAINFUL ARMS AND LEGS

You respond to a hotel near the airport for a man with generalised pain is his arms and legs; he is your first patient of the day. On arrival you are welcomed at the door by a hotel staff member who takes you to the patient's room, explaining to you that the patient called reception and in somewhat broken English requested a doctor, hence you were called.

Arriving in the room you are presented with an African man in his 40s, who is obviously in significant pain, and hands you what appears to be a note from a doctor or hospital that says: sickle cell disease.

What is sickle cell disease? Is this patient presenting in a typical way for this condition? What treatment, other than a thorough assessment, is of high priority here?

ANSWER & DISCUSSION

Sickle cell disease is an inherited condition that affects red blood cells, which causes them to change shape once they become deoxygenated, causing a half-moon shape, similar to a sickle, hence the name. These sickle cells often stick together, thus forming clot-like structures that can obstruct blood vessels and lead to episodes of severe pain (sickle cell crisis). The sickle cells also lead to lethargy and shortness of breath (due to decreased oxygen-carrying capability), pain in the arms, legs, sternum, spine, pelvis and abdomen, and increase the risk of strokes, regular infections, visual disturbances and myocardial infarctions. This patient is a typical presentation of sickle cell disease, because it mostly affects people of African, Caribbean, middle Eastern, eastern Mediterranean and Asian family background. Without the note from the patient and the language barrier, it would have been much harder to identify this condition.

The main treatment required is analgesia, as the pain can be debilitating. First-line options are paracetamol and non-steroidal anti-inflammatory drugs (NSAIDs), but very often this is not sufficient, making nitrous oxide and oxygen (Entonox), followed by oral morphine, the next best choices. Oxygen is not required by default and should only be administered if the patient is hypoxaemic.

CASE 82: BACK AND ABDOMINAL PAIN

During a nightshift you are sent to a 48-year-old female with back and abdominal pain that woke her up during the night. You arrive within 5 minutes of receiving the call. You and your colleague follow the patient into her living room where she explains that she has never had pain like this before, even during heavy periods. Initially she thought nothing of it, because she has been under a lot of stress and thought it might be indigestion. Vital signs and a history are taken, alongside a physical examination.

HR 98 beats/minute and regular

RR 20 breaths/minute

SpO_2 of 98% on room air

BP 90/50 mmHg

12-lead ECG showing a normal sinus rhythm

The physical examination reveals 8 out of 10 pain on the pain scale and a pulsatile, abdominal mass. No rebound tenderness is present. She has no allergies, takes ramipril once daily for hypertension, but has no other medical history. The pain started while she was asleep, so she does not know if the onset was sudden or got progressively worse.

What is the most likely diagnosis and what treatment is required?

ANSWER & DISCUSSION

This patient displays the classic signs of an abdominal aortic aneurysm (AAA) that may be close to rupture. These occur when the aorta dilates an additional 50% beyond its normal diameter, due to weakening of the arterial wall, leading to the pulsatile mass you palpated in her abdomen. Hypertension and family history are risk factors, but symptoms are often not present until rupture is imminent. Typical signs and symptoms are: sudden onset of pain in the back, abdomen, loin or groin, and a pulsatile mass. Signs of shock, such as hypotension and tachycardia or even bradycardia, are going to be present in patients where it has ruptured. Not all ruptured AAAs are equally likely to result in mortality, because it depends on size, location and time since it ruptured.

There is no pre-hospital specific treatment, other than early recognition, monitoring, obtaining intravenous access and rapid transportation to an appropriate facility, because these patients require imaging studies and urgent surgical repair.

CASE 83: HEADACHE

On a Sunday morning you are dispatched to Barbara, a 24-year-old pregnant female with a severe headache. After introducing yourself and gaining consent to assess her, your colleague obtains some vital signs before you proceed with history taking.

HR 94 beats/minute and regular

RR 18 breaths/minute

SpO_2 of 97% on room air

BP 150/90 mmHg

HGT 5.9 mmol/l

Temperature (tympanic) 36.9°C

12-lead ECG showing a normal sinus rhythm

Pain score for the headache of 6 out of 10

Allergies: None

Medication: Aspirin 70 mg once a day

Past medical history: First time pregnant, currently at 24 weeks' gestation with twins; GP told her she needs to come back every week for blood pressure checks, because her BP was apparently at risk of becoming quite high during pregnancy; no other medical or surgical history

Last meal/output: Breakfast 2 hours ago and urine output just thereafter

Events: She called 999 because her headache did not go away after a few hours and she is worried her BP might be the problem

Barbara most probably has which condition? What information other than the elevated BP is a contributing risk factor? Does this require an ED review?

ANSWER & DISCUSSION

Barbara is suffering from hypertension in pregnancy and is at particular risk for pre-eclampsia, which is defined as hypertension presenting without proteinuria after 20 weeks' gestation. Risk factors include first pregnancy and multiple pregnancy, in Barbara's case, as well as a being aged >40, chronic kidney disease, hypertension in previous pregnancies, diabetes and a pregnancy interval of more than 10 years.

Due to concerns about her blood pressure raised by her GP she has been prescribed 75 mg aspirin per day, which she should take until birth in an attempt to prevent progression to pre-eclampsia. Urine dipstick testing for proteinuria assessment should also be undertaken at regular intervals, but is not a necessary step to undertake for the ambulance service in a time of a hypertensive emergency, such as in this case.

The current blood pressure of 150/90 mmHg is considered moderate hypertension and requires hospital review in the ED today. Immediate medical advice should be sought even until the first 4 weeks postpartum if severe headaches, epigastric pain, vomiting, shortness of breath, or sudden swelling of face, hands or feet occurs.

Further resources/recommended reading

National Institute for Health and Care Excellence (2015) *Hypertension in Pregnancy*, London: NICE.

CASE 84: CONFUSION ON A CONSTRUCTION SITE

On a very warm summer's day during the mid-afternoon you are sent to a construction site for a man with acute-onset confusion. Less than 5 minutes after receiving the call you arrive on scene and are guided to a construction worker by his colleagues. Apparently their colleague Aiden started behaving oddly while they were paving the driveway, a project they had been working on for a few hours already, because they have a deadline to meet.

Aiden acknowledges your arrival and agrees to be assessed, but some interactions with you clearly highlight episodes of confusion.

Key findings from your assessment include the following:

He is alert, but intermittently confused

HR 106 beats/minute and regular

RR 22 breaths/minute

SpO_2 of 96% on room air

Temperature (tympanic) 39.8°C, but his skin appears dry

HGT 4.4 mmol/l

BP 95/60 mmHg

3-lead ECG showing sinus tachycardia (you have no 12-lead ECG available)

He is also complaining of nausea, but there is no evidence of vomiting present, denies any allergies and his colleagues are not aware of any medical problems that Aiden has.

What is the likely diagnosis?

What treatment is required?

ANSWER & DISCUSSION

Heat stroke is the most likely diagnosis, and the environment and setting of the incident provide numerous clues towards making this diagnosis: a very warm summer's day, the patient doing hard manual labour outside and possibly pushing himself harder than normal due to a looming deadline. Combining this with the vital signs and presentation, this diagnosis becomes even more likely.

Key features of heat stroke may include:

- A high body temperature (≥40°C, but Aiden is borderline);
- Hot and dry skin (perspiration limited due to dehydration);
- Tachycardia;
- Tachypnoea;
- Dizziness, nausea, vomiting;
- Confusion or unconsciousness.

Treatment should start with removal of the patient from the hot environment. Moving Aiden into the shade is an option, but an air-conditioned environment is preferable. Vital sign monitoring should be maintained throughout and oxygen should be administered if Aiden becomes hypoxaemic. Rehydration with oral fluids and/or intravenous 0.9% sodium chloride is urgently required and blood glucose control is also essential. Be careful about rehydrating at excessive speeds because vomiting may be the consequence. Aiden should be taken to hospital for review and a 12-lead ECG is also essential, in case any dysrhythmias are present that cannot be identified on a 3-lead ECG.

CASE 85: MOTORBIKE COLLISION

You are supporting a motor cross race together with a whole medical team when one rider misjudges a corner, crashes and gets flung into a tree next to the track. The race is stopped and you arrive at the patient's side within 60 seconds of the incident.

The 22-year-old patient is not showing signs of catastrophic haemorrhage, is alert and clearly breathing at a rate of approximately 20 breaths/minute. You palpate a radial pulse at 90 beats/minute and get one of your colleagues to maintain in-line c-spine stabilisation. As you progress through your assessments and alert the helicopter emergency medical services (HEMS) to facilitate more advanced care and transportation by air to the nearest major trauma centre, the patient is starting to become agitated and uncooperative due to his suspected traumatic brain injury.

Once you have established intravenous access, the only vital signs you have managed to assess for a second time are: RR of 20 breaths/minute, HR of 90 beats/minute, SpO_2 of 98% on oxygen, and pupils that are reactive to light at 4 mm on the left and 6 mm on the right side, when he starts pulling his oxygen mask off and attempts to get up and walk away. Despite three members of the medical team attempting to hold him back, you can barely keep him under control.

Which pharmacological option is available to you to manage this agitation/combativeness from the suspected head injury?

ANSWER & DISCUSSION

A patient with traumatic brain injury may become agitated and combative, thereby making it impossible to ensure effective oxygenation. In such cases midazolam administration may be warranted, especially where other attempts to ensure effective patient management and oxygenation, such as verbal de-escalation, have not worked. In patients aged <60 years, 0.5–1.0 mg can be administered every 2 minutes up to a maximum dose of 7.5 mg. This will allow for facilitation of effective treatment and oxygenation, and will also buy time until the HEMS team arrives, because head injury patients often require drug-facilitated intubation.

CASE 86: DISCOLOURED STOOLS

You are working a weekend shift at the local walk-in treatment centre when you are assigned to assess a 47-year-old male with discoloured stools. He explains to you that he has been noticing the black discoloration over the last 2 days and has been feeling particularly tired for about the same length of time. Before you assess any vital signs you perform an abdominal exam and discover epigastric tenderness and he tells you that he thinks he may have an ulcer, because his GP once mentioned something about it, but he cannot remember the details (i.e. he has one or if he is at risk for one) as it was 'absolutely ages ago'.

His vital signs are as follows:

HR 88 beats/minute

RR 16 breaths/minute

BP 145/80 mmHg

Temperature (tympanic) 37.0°C

He has no allergies and occasionally takes ibuprofen and paracetamol for back pain.

What can cause the discoloration?

Is there any further information about the stool that would help you diagnose the condition?

ANSWER & DISCUSSION

The colour of a stool can be affected by various things, including blood from the gastrointestinal (GI) tract, iron supplements or even eating significant amounts of liquorice. Knowing about the consistency of the stool would be particularly beneficial, because, when stools are of tar-like consistency, it is a reliable indicator for upper GI tract bleeding. This patient requires various blood tests, including a full blood count, urea and electrolytes, liver function tests, a clotting profile and a referral for a review by a gastroenterologist, if there are no immediate concerns discovered. A quick visual inspection of the mucous membranes should also be undertaken, because a pale colour is an indication of anaemia, which could be a consequence of prolonged bleeding.

CASE 87: WALKING DOWN THE STREET IN HER PYJAMAS

On your way from hospital to your designated standby point at about 01:00 you and your colleague notice an elderly woman wearing pyjamas walking down the road. This does appear rather strange at this time of night, so you decide to inform the dispatcher of this and inform him that you are going to investigate and check if she requires any assistance.

You pull over and get out the ambulance and attempt to start a conversation with her by introducing yourself and asking her if she needed any help. She says her name is Jenny and that she is 'on her way somewhere'. This appears odd to you, so you ask her if she would like a lift, because she appears rather lost. She smiles vividly and thanks you for being 'such a kind person' and she sits down on the stretcher. As you help to buckle her seatbelt you notice a bracelet on her left arm that reads 'My name is Jennifer and I have dementia'. You spend a few minutes talking to her when she agrees to be assessed by you and you find no abnormalities of her vital signs. During the FAST exam she finds it difficult to follow the instructions, so you are unable to complete it properly.

When you mention the hospital name to her that you would like to take her to for further assessment and because you have no idea where she lives, she appears to recognise the name and happily agrees to be taken there.

Is this the appropriate decision?

ANSWER & DISCUSSION

Patients with dementia are often confused and may therefore not be able to provide you with a reliable or accurate history. Jennifer is convinced she is going somewhere in particular, but cannot explain where that place is, confirming that she is confused at this time. Her inability to concentrate on the tasks during the FAST exam are another symptom of dementia, but also raise the potential risk of not detecting an acute stroke by not being able to complete the exam. The time and place that she was picked up at do not give you the opportunity to obtain a history from carers, friends, family or even obtaining contact information from any paperwork or other documentation that would be present in Jennifer's home environment. This leaves little choices in terms of where to transport the patient to at this time and context, making ED the only viable option for Jennifer.

Further resources/recommended reading

Voss, S., Black, S., Brandling, J. et al. (2017) Home or hospital for people with dementia and one or more other multimorbidities: What is the potential to reduce avoidable emergency admissions? The HOMEWARD Project Protocol, *BMJ Open*, 7(4), e016651.

CASE 88: MUSCULAR PAIN

A 28-year-old female with severe muscular pain in her right thigh has called 999, after the pain became progressively worse over the last few hours. Your assessment of her vital signs and history reveals the following:

HR 88 beats/minute and regular

RR 18 breaths/minute

SpO_2 of 98% on room air

BP 125/78 mmHg

Temperature (tympanic) 36.9°C

HGT 6.1 mmol/l

12-lead ECG showing normal sinus rhythm

Allergies: Peanuts

Medication: EpiPen® for her peanut allergy

Past medical history: Twisted ankle a year ago from falling on the treadmill; no allergic reaction to peanuts in over 5 years now

Last meal/output: Pasta with pesto for lunch about an hour ago; urine appeared very dark when she urinated about 40 minutes ago

Events: She developed pain in her right thigh after returning from her morning work-out and it got progressively worse

Physical assessment of her right thigh reveals tenderness and pain, and when she walked to the door to let you in she said she felt like she had less power in the left leg than normal.

What condition is she suffering from?

What treatment is required and can she be treated at home?

ANSWER & DISCUSSION

This patient is suffering from exertional rhabdomyolysis, which refers to rhabdomyolysis caused by strenuous exercise, such as found in CrossFit, a type of high-intensity workout regimen that has gained worldwide popularity. Rhabdomyolysis occurs when striated skeletal muscle breaks down and necrosis occurs, leading to pain and swelling. Once the intracellular content of the dead cells is released into the bloodstream, it can lead to an acute kidney injury, thus causing the discoloured urine (caused by myoglobin and often described as tea coloured). Hyperthermia and dehydration, as may be experienced during strenuous and prolonged exercise, are both considered contributing factors to rhabdomyolysis. Mild cases can be treated with rest and oral rehydration. This patient does, however, require hospital admission to check creatine kinase (CK) levels to confirm the diagnosis and initiate treatment. CK levels should be 5–10 times the normal limit and be present with the associated symptoms mentioned above to confirm the diagnosis. Treatment has to include intravenous fluid administration of 0.9% sodium chloride (1–2 l/h to treat dehydration). The aim is to maintain urine output at around 200 ml/h, and further treatment may be required if this cannot be achieved, but diuretics should not be used.

Further resources/recommended reading

Tietze, D. and Borchers, J. (2014) Exertional rhabdomyolysis in the athlete: a clinical review, *Sports Health: A Multidisciplinary Approach*, 6(4), 336–339.

CASE 89: ANIMAL BITE

Your ambulance is sent to a 72-year-old female who sustained an animal bite from her cat. Emily, your patient, meets you at the door, pressing a partially blood-soaked tea towel on to her left arm. She explains to you that she was concerned about her cat because she was walking differently from normal. However, when she picked the cat up to assess her, she lashed out with her claws and bit Emily in the lower left arm, causing bleeding and pain. Your assessment of Emily's vital signs reveals no abnormalities other than a slightly irregular radial pulse and the ECG shows a sinus rhythm with atrial fibrillation. The physical assessment of the wound shows some skin lacerations from the cat's claws and very small punctures from her teeth, as well. The bleeding has stopped already, so there is no immediate need to apply pressure dressings.

Emily's history is as follows:

Allergies: None

Medication: Warfarin

Past medical history: Atrial fibrillation

Last meal/output: Breakfast 2 hours ago; urine output normal, bowels opened after breakfast

Events: Tried to pick up her cat to assess the observed limp and was scratched and bitten when she did so

What underlying structures may be damaged by cat bites?

What other considerations are there with cat bites?

Why has Emily suffered from quite significant bleeding from a fairly small injury?

ANSWER & DISCUSSION

Cat bites, although looking less dramatic than most dog bites, tend to penetrate deeper into the tissue due to their sharper, finer teeth. This may lead to penetration of joints, tendons and bones, and also introduce saliva deep into the wound(s), increasing the risk of further complications, such as infections. Tetanus vaccination status should be assessed and may require a booster, particularly if the tetanus risk is increased (e.g. foreign bodies in the wound or a delay of more than 6 hours since the incident occurred). The reason Emily was bleeding significantly, i.e. enough to leave her tea towel visibly soaked, is due to her regular medication, warfarin. As it is an anticoagulant, it increases the risk of bleeding and therefore also affects how long it takes bleeding to stop. On a patient who is not on warfarin this bleeding may have been hardly noticeable and probably not lead to such distinct skin lacerations.

Further resources/recommended reading

National Institute for Health and Care Excellence (2018) *Bites—Human and animal*, London: NICE.

CASE 90: INTRAOSSEOUS ACCESS

During the resuscitation of a 56-year-old male you are in charge of vascular access and drug administration, while the rest of the team manages the chest compressions, airway and breathing. After two unsuccessful attempts at intravenous cannulation you change your approach by selecting intraosseous (IO) access as the alternative. The equipment you are issued with today includes three types of IO needles (15 mm, 25 mm and 45 mm in length), the IO driver, securing device and all other necessary accessories.

Depending on the type of IO device, common landmarks in adult patients may include:

- Proximal humerus (humeral head);
- Proximal tibia;
- Distal tibia;
- (Sternum, with specialised, selected devices).

You clean the insertion site and are just about to start the procedure when you start thinking about the next steps you need to undertake. The most common indication for obtaining IO access is the inability to obtain intravenous access after multiple, unsuccessful attempts, but what are the contraindications? What if you are not able to aspirate bone marrow. Does this mean the procedure failed?

ANSWER & DISCUSSION

Intraosseous access has become a common route of vascular access within the civilian ambulance service setting over recent years and is not just typical in paediatric patients. Contraindications, however obvious, need to be considered for all procedures and may include:

- Inability to identify the landmarks (e.g. due to overlying tissue or large muscular mass);
- Fracture of the selected extremity (or sternum);
- Infection of the proposed insertion site;
- History of significant orthopaedic procedure at the proposed insertion site (e.g. joint replacement, prosthetic limb, prosthetic joint);
- Less than 48 hours have passed since IO access was last performed in the selected bone (successful or unsuccessful).

If you are unable to aspirate bone marrow after the insertion of the IO needle, then this does not mean that the procedure failed. Continue with the 0.9% sodium chloride flush (5–10 ml in adults) and consider aspirating afterwards to confirm that the IO needle has been inserted into the bone marrow. Remember to write the date and time of insertion an any supplied bands/labels to ensure that IO access is not attempted again within the next 48–72 hours (depending on your local guidelines).

CASE 91: WHITE MAGIC

During the early hours of a Saturday morning you are working alone on a rapid response vehicle (RRV) and are dispatched to an 18-year-old male who appears hyperactive to his flatmates. They show you into the lounge where Craig is nervously pacing the length of the room. They tell you that he came back from a party with his classmates from university and that he has been hyperactive since then, and that his knuckles are all bruised, scratched and look like he hit something or someone. You introduce yourself and Craig immediately strikes up a conversation with you. To reduce the risk to yourself you ensure that there is an easily identifiable escape route available for Craig, in case he starts to feel uneasy or gets aggressive. During the conversation you establish that he went out with his classmates to celebrate passing his first-ever university assignment and that one of them gave him some crystal type-looking powder called 'white magic' that he then swallowed. He said he felt really energised, but that feeling is not going away now.

He agrees to have his vital signs taken, but you only manage to obtain a partial history:

HR 126 beats/minute and regular

RR 22 breaths/minute

SpO_2 of 96% on room air

HGT 5.2 mmol/l

Temperature (tympanic) 37.6°C

3-lead ECG showing sinus tachycardia (patient too agitated to obtain a clear 12-lead ECG tracing)

History reveals no allergies and no regular medication, but Craig does not answer any of the other questions, because he keeps on pacing around the room.

What is white magic? Which class of drug did he most probably ingest? What treatment is needed?

ANSWER & DISCUSSION

White magic is a street name for a version of synthetic cathinone drugs, often referred to as bath salts. These can be taken orally, crushed and snorted, smoked or injected, and are categorised as amphetamines. Sympathomimetic toxicity is the result, leading to euphoria, agitation and tremors, tachycardia and hypertension. Higher doses can cause seizures, intracranial haemorrhage and cardiovascular complications (e.g. myocardial infarction, ventricular dysrhythmias).

Treatment has to address certain key areas, particularly hyperthermia and dehydration, because persistent hyperthermia is associated with increased morbidity and mortality. Agitation and seizures should both be managed with benzodiazepines, such as diazepam or midazolam, depending on local guidelines. Hypoglycaemia is always a concern in agitated patients, as in this case, because persistent agitation can lead to a failure to hydrate and eat, putting Craig at higher risk for hypoglycaemia. Transport to the ED is required, because the toxic effects of amphetamines cannot be clearly predicted, as dosages and strengths of ingredients are not clearly defined or regulated. Cardiovascular effects can be long lasting and significant, making continuous ECG monitoring essential.

CASE 92: 'THE BABY IS COMING'

You are first on scene as a lone responder on a rapid response vehicle of a maternity call for a 29-year-old female in labour. Apparently the contractions are about 5 minutes apart and no ambulance is currently available to provide transportation. You take all your medical equipment into the house, as well as a maternity pack, a blanket and a suction unit. You conduct a thorough assessment and find the following:

HR 110 beats/minute and regular

RR 20 breaths/minute

BP 140/90 mmHg

Temperature (tympanic) 37.0°C

HGT 6.2 mmol/l

History about the pregnancy

- Week 40 of pregnancy;
- Gravida 5, parity 4 (fifth pregnancy, four previous births);
- Water broke about 15 minutes ago;
- Umbilical cord physically visible as a large loop.

Allergies: Penicillin

Medication: Omeprazole

Past medical history: Gastric reflux during pregnancy

Last meal/output: Lunch 2 hours ago; urine and bowel movements normal

Events: Her waters broke about 15 minutes ago so she called 999, because she needs help to get to hospital and some of the umbilical cord was visible between her legs; all her children are with her in the house, but no other adult

What treatments are specifically needed for prolapsed umbilical cord presentation? Are there any other considerations that you need to make provisions for?

ANSWER & DISCUSSION

The biggest danger in this scenario is fetal asphyxia caused by compression of the umbilical cord and arterial vasospasm due to the colder, outside, ambient air, thus preventing blood flow to and from the fetus. Due to this mechanism cord compression needs to be prevented through manual interventions. In cases where only a small section is showing, ambulance crews may undertake one attempt to gently push it back into the vagina with two fingers, but this would not be possible in this case. Large loops of umbilical cord need to be covered in dry padding to avoid further exposure to the cooler environment and the mother needs to be placed in the left lateral position with padding under her hips to aid reduction of pressure on the cord. Nitrous oxide and oxygen (Entonox) may be administered to reduce the urge to push, thus delaying the delivery as much as possible. Intravenous access should be obtained as soon as practicable, but as you are awaiting the arrival of an ambulance you might have sufficient time before departure to do this, otherwise do it en route. Her children are all with her in the house, but as there is no adult to look after them you need to make provisions with family or neighbours to look after them once you depart for the nearest ED. A pre-alert and blue light transportation are essential.

CASE 93: DIFFICULTY BREATHING

You are called as an emergency to a 6-month-old male whose parents are concerned because he seems to be finding it difficult to breathe. On arrival you are presented with a child who appears slightly pale, is displaying nasal flaring when breathing and is alert. The mother explains that he has had a cold for about 2 days with a dry cough and runny nose; 2 hours ago the symptoms got much worse and his breathing worsened. The patient has not had any significant illnesses before and has never had anything like this. The last 2 days he has been feeding well and his nappies have been wet, but today he is not feeding and seems agitated.

You expose the chest and identify intercostal recession. On auscultation you hear a global expiratory wheeze. You take the following vital signs:

RR 50 breaths/minute

HR 150 beats/minute

SpO_2 91% on room air

Temperature (tympanic) 37.9°C

What is the likely diagnosis?

ANSWER & DISCUSSION

The patient is presenting with bronchiolitis. This is a viral infection of the small airways that affects young children, particularly those younger than 1 year. The severity of the illness is dictated by the severity of the symptoms; in this case, the patient is hypoxic and using accessory muscles to breathe, which indicates severe dyspnoea.

The patient should receive supportive oxygen and transportation to hospital. Although there is a wheeze, nebulised salbutamol has not been shown to affect outcomes so should not normally be used if you are relatively confident in your diagnosis of bronchiolitis. Bronchiolitis is a viral infection so antibiotics are not required. If the patient meets all of the green criteria on the NICE traffic light system then it may be appropriate to discharge the patient at scene with thorough safety netting advice. An overview of risk factors and features of severe illness can be seen in Figure 2.5.

Further resources/recommended reading

National Institute for Health and Care Excellence (2015) *Bronchiolitis in Children*, London: NICE.

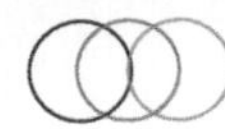

Risk level	Features
High	Ashen, blue or mottled appearance Unresponsive, difficult or impossible to rouse Appears unwell Moderate/severe sternal or intercostal recession Profound tachypnoea Other red flags associated with serious illness (e.g. symptoms of meningitis, sepsis, focal neurological symptoms)
Intermediate	Pale Lethargic Not interacting normally Nasal flaring Oxygen saturations <95% Tachypnoeic Crackles on auscultation
Low	Well perfused Interacting normally Crying normally Perfused and moist mucosa No intermediate or high level risk features of severe illness present

Figure 2.5 Risk levels and features of severe illness

CASE 94: CRICKET PLAYER WITH A HEAD INJURY

You are called to a cricket pitch for a player who has sustained a head injury and is unconscious. En route you are told by control that HEMS are aware of this call and would like you to update them when you are on scene. On arrival you are told that a batsman, who was not wearing a helmet, was hit in the head by the cricket ball and collapsed. As you approach the patient your primary survey reveals that he is unresponsive, looks pale and is breathing. You ask your crewmate to take some vital signs as you begin to assess the patient's head.

HR 85 beats/minute

RR 12 breaths/minute

BP 179/110 mmHg

GCS 3/15

ECG showing normal sinus rhythm

On examination of the head you see a depressed skull fracture near to the left temple. You do not identify any other injuries on your secondary survey.

HEMS want an update. What do you tell them?

What is the appropriate treatment and destination for this patient?

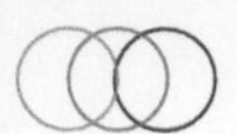

ANSWER & DISCUSSION

The patient has sustained a serious isolated head injury and it is likely that he has a traumatic brain injury that requires treatment at a major trauma centre. First, you need to consider how far the major trauma centre is by road and how long it would take HEMS to get to you. The other consideration is what skills HEMS can bring to the scene. This patient is a candidate for undergoing rapid sequence induction to protect his airway and regulate ventilation to reduce secondary brain damage. Traumatic brain injuries can be categorised as primary and secondary brain injury. Primary brain injuries occur at the moment of impact and paramedics can do nothing about this damage. Secondary brain injury is that injury arising from subsequent hypoxia, hypercapnia and other symptoms that damage the brain. The mainstay of immediate treatment is adequate airway management and oxygenation to protect the brain as much as possible, which is optimised by rapid sequence induction. Both the HEMS team and the major trauma centre can provide this, so you need to weigh up the quickest way for the patient to receive this intervention.

HEMS tell you that they can be on scene within 15 minutes and your nearest major trauma centre is 20 minutes away, so you decide to convey this patient to hospital in your ambulance.

You should not delay on scene time with this patient. It is reasonable to aim for a scene time of less than 10 minutes. Your priority is simple airway management and oxygenation. An oropharyngeal or nasopharyngeal airway is appropriate with 15 l/min of oxygen to try to minimise secondary brain injury. Hyper- or hypoventilation should be avoided so, if the patient's respiratory rate falls and you need to assist ventilation, this should be done at the normal rate and depth.

CASE 95: DOG BITE

You are working in a minor injuries unit and are presented with a 34-year-old male who has been bitten by a dog. He pulls down his trousers to reveal two puncture wounds on his right upper thigh, which have been caused by the dog's teeth. The wounds are not actively bleeding but they have clearly penetrated down to the subcutaneous layer and you can see fatty tissue. He is in a small amount of pain, has not taken any analgesia and has sustained no other injuries.

What is you management of this patient?

ANSWER & DISCUSSION

First, simple analgesia can be given following the WHO pain ladder; paracetamol is an appropriate choice. The mouths of animals have millions of bacteria in them and therefore bite wounds are at particularly high risk of bacterial infection. Therefore wounds around joints and other underlying structures are of particular concern. This wound is on the patient's thigh where there is a lot of fatty tissue. The wound is deep and would usually require closing, but closing the wound now would create the perfect anaerobic environment for bacteria to thrive and cause an infection. Therefore, the wound should be irrigated thoroughly and dressed with a view to reassessing the wound in 48 hours and allowing the wound to heal naturally.

Antibiotics could be given prophylactically because of the high risk of infection. This is controversial and a more conservative approach would be to reassess the wound after 48 hours and only administer antibiotics if there are signs of an infection. You should consider infection if the wound is red, excessive pus comes from the wound and/or it is hot to touch.

You should ensure that the patient has adequate tetanus cover and provide a tetanus vaccination if not. You should also consider the risk of rabies; although there is low incidence in the UK, you should consider and document this.

Further resources/recommended reading

National Institute for Health and Care Excellence (2018) *Bites—Human and animal*, London: NICE.

CASE 96: BACK PAIN

It is 03:00 and you are called to a 58-year-old female complaining of back pain. Upon arrival her husband tells you that she awoke in the middle of the night, rolled over to get out of bed and experienced excruciating lower back pain. She has never had back pain like this before, but does report that she has been spending more time in bed due to illness recently.

You primary survey reveals no concerns and you can see that the patient is in a lot of pain. You take the following history:

HPC: Woke up, rolled over in bed and experienced severe lower back pain

S—across the whole of the lower back and her neck feels stiff

O—20 minutes ago when she woke up

C—sharp in nature

R—radiates across whole back

A—feels slightly nauseous, stiff neck, back feels tight

T—constant pain

E—moving makes it worse, staying still helps

S—9/10

PMH: Breast cancer, had mastectomy 5 months ago

DHx: Undergoing chemotherapy; last had it 2 weeks ago

SHx: Lives with husband; she is usually quite independent but the last few weeks has been in bed much more

FHx: Nothing significant

RoS: She has not been incontinent

Are there any red flags with this patient?

What would be your management?

ANSWER & DISCUSSION

In some ways this case sounds like muscular back pain. It was caused by rolling over, the patient has been increasingly bed bound and the nature of the pain suggests that it could be muscular. However, the patient is undergoing chemotherapy for cancer and this is a red flag for sudden back pain. It could suggest that the cancer has metastasized in the spine and impinged on the spinal cord causing spinal cord compression. Back pain such as this can be the first sign that the cancer has metastasized and it can cause irreversible damage if not treated quickly.

This patient requires hospitalisation for an MRI scan to investigate the cause of the back pain and rule out serious pathology. In the meantime, analgesia should be given because the patient is scoring her pain at 9/10. It would be appropriate to obtain intravenous access and administer intravenous paracetamol and/or morphine.

Further resources/recommended reading

National Institute for Health and Care Excellence (2008) *Metastatic Spinal Cord Compression in Adults: Risk assessment, diagnosis and management*, London: NICE.

CASE 97: POSSIBLE STROKE

You are working on an RRV and are called to a 76-year-old female who is having symptoms of a stroke. You arrive at the patient's house quickly and, as you are walking up the stairs, her husband explains that the patient suddenly started slurring her words and he couldn't understand what she was saying. In the bedroom you introduce yourself to the patient and she acknowledges you. The primary survey reveals no deficits and, as you speak to the patient, you do not notice slurred speech. The husband explains that it has gotten much better and her speech is back to normal. He wonders if he had misunderstood what was going on or imagined the symptoms. You ask him how long the symptoms were present before he phoned for an ambulance and he says 15 minutes. Her vital signs are as follows:

RR 18 breaths/minute

HR 80 beats/minute

HGT 5.6 mmol/l

BP 137/78 mmHg

PERRL 4 mm

FAST negative

What is the likely diagnosis?

What can help to guide your management of this patient?

ANSWER & DISCUSSION

This patient was having one of the signs of a stroke but it resolved within 20 minutes. Therefore, this is a transient ischaemic attack (TIA), colloquially called a mini-stroke. The definition of a TIA is when a patient has signs of a stroke but they fully resolve spontaneously within 24 hours. A TIA does not cause lasting damage. However, a TIA is often a precursor to a stroke, indicating that there is significant atherosclerosis in the cerebral arteries. Therefore, although the symptoms are now fully resolved for the patient, it is important to act proactively and aggressively to try to prevent the patient from having a stroke.

The ABCD2 score can be used to assess the risk of a patient going on to have a stroke, and therefore can guide your decision-making on the safety of discharging this patient at scene. The ABCD2 score takes into account age, blood pressure, clinical features, duration of symptoms and history of diabetes. This patient scores 3 and is therefore considered to be a lower risk for having a stoke. Patients who have a TIA should start taking aspirin immediately and an appointment should be made for them at the TIA clinic within the next 48 hours. You may be able to do this directly through an agreed pathway or you may need to contact the patient's GP to arrange this. Had the patient scored more than 3 on the ABCD2 score then it would be appropriate to convey her to hospital due to the risk of having a stroke.

Further resources/recommended reading

National Institute for Health and Care Excellence (2017) *Stroke and TIA*, London: NICE.

CASE 98: DOCTOR'S NOTES

During transportation of a patient from a GP surgery to the ED you have some time available to read the referral letter that was given to you for the receiving facility. The letter reads as follows:

> Thank you for seeing my patient Mr Julian Smith (52-year-old male) at such short notice. He presented to my surgery multiple times over the last month for a recurring cough that has since progressed to produce discoloured sputum. Medication he has received so far: amoxicillin 500 mg tds 5/7; paracetamol 1 g qds, all of which initially resolved the symptoms. Now c/o the same type of cough again. O/A in my surgery today he was short of breath and he was LIC of ambulance crew for transportation to ED at 15:22, after a thorough assessment.
>
> I would appreciate it if the following investigations could be undertaken in your ED and you could send me the report:
>
> CXR, FBC, U&Es and CRP.
>
> Kind regards,
>
> Doctor Carrington

What do all these abbreviations mean?

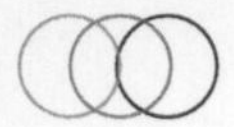

ANSWER & DISCUSSION

Amoxicillin 500 mg tds 5/7: take this antibiotic three times a day for 5 days

Paracetamol 1 g qds: take 1 g of paracetamol four times a day

C/O stands for complaining of

O/A stands for on arrival

LIC stands for left in care of

CXR: chest X-ray

FBC: full blood count

U&Es: urea and electrolytes

CRP: C-reactive protein

CASE 99: 'HE IS NOT MOVING HIS ARM'

You are working on the RRV and are called to a 2-year-old male who is not moving his arm. His mother tells you that she has noticed her son has been more subdued than normal, and is holding his right arm by his side and not moving it. On examination you note that there is no deformity or swelling to the arm and no pain on palpation. However, when you attempt to move the child's arm he is in a lot of pain. There are no other injuries or issues so you ask the mother if there is anything the child has done that could have caused an arm injury. The only thing she can think of is that they have been playing in the park today and they were swinging him around a lot by his arms, although she does not remember him injuring it specifically.

What would be your primary diagnosis?

What would be your management?

ANSWER & DISCUSSION

The patient has most probably suffered a pulled elbow. This is a subluxation of the radial head through the annular ligament, usually caused by a sudden pull on the child's arm. In this case swinging the patient by his arms could have caused this injury. Children with a pulled elbow most commonly present with limited pain but unable to move their arm.

You have assessed the rest of the arm and not found any significant injuries or pain, so you can be fairly confident in your diagnosis of pulled elbow, and it would be appropriate to attempt to relocate it using either a pronation or supination manoeuvre. The pronation method requires you to press the child's radial head while pronating the forearm as far as it will go, then flexing the elbow. The supination method requires you to supinate the forearm and then flex the elbow. If the radial head relocates then you may feel a 'pop', and the child should be able to use his arm again without any pain.

If there is doubt about the diagnosis, or the manoeuvres are unsuccessful, then the child will require transportation to hospital for further investigation. It is also important to consider the possibility of a non-accidental injury, so a good history is important to ensure that the mechanisms described match the injury. Similarly, it is good practice to check previous healthcare contacts if you have the ability to do so, in order to take note of any patterns of injury occurring.

CASE 100: LOSS OF VISION

You are working in a minor injuries unit and are presented with a 57-year-old male who is complaining of visual problems. He tells you that he was walking the dog earlier in the day when he started seeing floaters in his vision. He thought nothing of it until he was at home and started experiencing the feeling of flashing lights. The flashing lights would come episodically, lasting around 30 seconds. He took a taxi to the minor injuries unit because he could not see well enough to drive, and he now reports that there is a black patch at the top of his vision. He has not had any trauma to the eye and has never experienced anything like this before.

What is the most likely diagnosis?

What is the correct management plan?

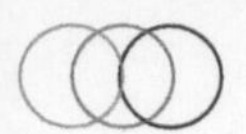

ANSWER & DISCUSSION

This patient is displaying common signs of a detached retina. As the retina starts to detach, floaters are seen in the vision as blood and pigment cells cast shadows on the retina. Further detachment causes flashes of light and eventually visual loss, often described as a curtain coming down over the vision. Visual loss is a symptom that indicates the level of retinal detachment is severe and warrants immediate assessment and treatment by an ophthalmologist to save his vision.

In such an obvious and severe case of retinal detachment it is not necessary to carry out further tests; however, when more subtle you can check visual fields and visual acuity to identify visual problems. It would be pertinent to identify which eye has been affected and this can be done simply by covering up one eye at a time to see which one has the symptoms. It would be appropriate to contact ophthalmology to refer your patient straight to them and arrange transport to hospital.

Further resources/recommendations

National Institute for Health and Care Excellence (2015) *Retinal Detachment*, London: NICE.

INDEX

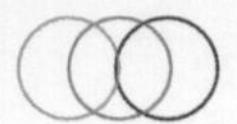

 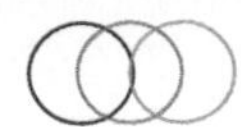

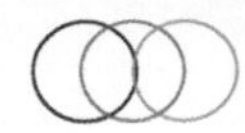